Risking Your Health

HUMAN DEVELOPMENT PERSPECTIVES

Risking Your Health

Causes, Consequences, and Interventions to Prevent Risky Behaviors

Damien de Walque, Editor

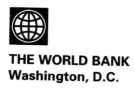

THE WORLD BANK
Washington, D.C.

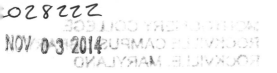

Contents

Maps

Tables

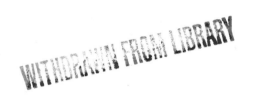

Foreword

A growing share of the burden of disease across the world is associated with risky behaviors by individuals. Drug use, smoking, alcohol, unhealthy eating causing obesity, and unsafe sex are highly prevalent in low-income countries, even though they are traditionally associated with richer countries. In some cases like smoking and obesity, the prevalence in developing countries is growing at an alarming rate.

The consequences of risky behaviors are rarely limited to the individuals engaging in them. In certain cases the link is direct: drug consumption, smoking, alcohol use, poor diet, and HIV and sexually transmitted infections among mothers have detrimental impacts on the fetus, secondhand smoke is recognized as a serious health hazard, and unprotected sex and needle sharing lead to the transmission of HIV and other sexually transmitted infections. In other cases, the links are less direct but not necessarily less real: the long-term health consequences of many of these behaviors are costly to treat and could stretch households' finances and worsen poverty. Finally, these risky behaviors have consequences for society as a whole since they often trigger a nontrivial amount of public health expenditures and lead to declines in aggregate productivity through premature death and morbidity.

Understanding the factors driving those behaviors, their incidence, and consequences, and the effectiveness of policies and programs to affect them in a sustainable way, represents a priority not only from a public health perspective but from a broader development one.

This volume represents an important contribution to fill the knowledge gap in this area. Following on the steps of the previous volumes in the Human Development Perspectives series, it summarizes the existing evidence about the causes and consequences of those behaviors, as well as about interventions aimed at preventing them from a broad range of sources.

Quite often, smoking, obesity, risky sex, and drug or alcohol use are analyzed separately. One of the contributions of this book is to regroup the analysis of those behaviors under the same conceptual framework, stressing their common features. It brings together perspectives from various disciplines while using an economic framework to ground the consideration of public policies. Through its review of the international evidence, the volume provides extremely useful insights into the design of public policies. It shows, for example, that public health interventions via legislation with strong enforcement mechanisms can be more effective than simple communication campaigns informing consumers about the risks associated with certain behaviors, since translating knowledge into concrete changes in behavior seems to be hard to achieve. It also shows that economic mechanisms such as taxes (especially on alcohol and tobacco products), subsidies (such as free condoms), and conditional/unconditional cash transfers can be used to reduce risky behaviors (for example, in HIV prevention), with some successes.

This volume should serve to encourage a fruitful exchange between public health experts, economists, and policy makers to inform public policies in an area of growing importance across the world.

Ariel Fiszbein
Chief Economist for Human Development
Chair, Editorial Board, Human Development Perspectives series
World Bank
Washington, D.C.

Acknowledgments

The authors would like to convey their deep gratitude to Ariel Fiszbein for his leadership and guidance throughout the entire production of this book, from suggesting its realization to following and guiding closely each of the steps. Nicole Klingen and Adam Wagstaff also provided very useful guidance and comments.

John Cawley, Markus Goldstein, Albertus Voetberg, and Abdo Yazbeck have been outstanding peer reviewers, careful, attentive, and constructive from the concept note stage to the final version. We are also very grateful for the very useful comments received from Omar Arias, María Eugenia Bonilla-Chacín, Leslie Elder, Margaret Grosh, Patricio V. Marquez, Andre Medici, Montserrat Meiro-Lorenzo, Maryse Pierre-Louis, Claudia Rokx, and Eileen Sullivan.

Alexandra Melo provided outstanding research assistance. Paola Scalabrin, Mary C. Fisk, Barbara Hart, and Linda Stringer greatly improved the manuscript thanks to their editorial assistance and guidance. Jeffrey Lecksell and Alexandra Melo expertly designed the maps used in this volume. Susheela Jonnakuty and Zaure Schwade offered excellent support during the production of this volume.

This book received generous financial support from the Spanish Impact Evaluation Fund (SIEF).

About the Authors

Damien de Walque is a senior economist in the Development Research Group (Human Development and Public Services Team) at the World Bank. He received his PhD in Economics from the University of Chicago in 2003. His research interests include health and education and the interactions between them. He has an extensive expertise in HIV/AIDS and smoking-related projects and a large number of publications, both in economics and the medical literature. He is working on evaluating the impact of HIV/AIDS interventions and policies in several Sub-Saharan African countries. His current work is focused on evaluating the impact of financial incentives on health and education outcomes.

Alaka Holla is an economist in the Chief Economist's Office of the World Bank's Human Development Network. Her research focuses on measuring the relationships among prices, access, and quality in health and education markets in low-income settings. She is currently contributing to analytical work in Argentina, India, Kosovo, Nigeria, and Tanzania; in the coming year, she will be part of the team writing the *World Development Report 2015*, which will focus on the behavioral and social foundations of development. She holds a PhD in Economics from Brown University.

Mattias Lundberg is Senior Economist in the Social Protection and Labor Team at the World Bank and is the World Bank's Focal Point on Youth. He is the director of the Global Program on Youth Employment, and he manages experiments in labor market programs for youth under the Strategic

Impact Evaluation Fund and the Adolescent Girls' Initiative. He was one of the authors of the *World Development Report 2007: Development and the Next Generation*. His most recent book (2012) is on the impact of economic crises on households and children; his other research encompasses income distribution, public services, HIV/AIDS, and other topics.

Aakanksha (Aaka) H. Pande is a health economist at the World Bank, where she specializes in health nutrition and population issues in the Middle East and North Africa. She focuses on the evaluation of health sector programs on which she has worked in India, Mexico, Pakistan, and Sri Lanka. Her work has been published in peer-reviewed academic journals and mainstream media like the *New York Times*. She holds a PhD in Evaluative Sciences and Statistics of Health Policy from Harvard University, a Master's in Global Health and Population from the Harvard School of Public Health, a Fellowship in Global Health from Cambridge University, and a Bachelor's in Science in Molecular Biology from Yale University.

Sébastien Piguet is a student in Economics at the Paris School of Economics and at Ecole Normale Supérieure; he specialized in Health Economics. He spent the academic year 2011–12 at Cornell University as a visiting student in the department of Economics and the department of Human Ecology. He worked as a consultant for the World Bank from May to September 2012. His previous publications include articles about French and European public policies in *Année politique, économique et sociale* and *Chantiers politiques*.

Gil Shapira is an economist in the Development Research Group (Human Development and Public Services Team) of the World Bank. His work focuses on analyzing demographic and health issues in developing countries, with an emphasis on Sub-Saharan Africa. More specifically, he studies decision making in the context of the HIV/AIDS epidemic, the transition from adolescence to adulthood in Malawi, and the impact of interventions to improve maternal and child health in different countries. He received his PhD in Economics from the University of Pennsylvania.

Abbreviations

ACE	Adverse Childhood Events study
AIDS	acquired immunodeficiency syndrome
ART	anti-retroviral therapy
ATS	amphetamine-type stimulants
BMI	body mass index
CCTs	conditional cash transfers
CM	contingency management
COPD	chronic obstructive pulmonary disorder
CVD	cardiovascular disease
DBM	Double Burden of Malnutrition
FCTC	Framework Convention for Tobacco Control
GDP	Gross Domestic Product
GISAH	Global Information System on Alcohol and Health
HIV	human immunodeficiency virus
HSV–2	herpes-simplex virus–type 2
IEC	information and communication campaigns
INCA	Instituto Nacional de Câncer
NCDs	noncommunicable diseases
NSPs	needle and syringe exchange programs
OECD	Organisation for Economic Co-operation and Development
PDS	patterns of drinking score
SIEF	Spanish Impact Evaluation Fund
STI	sexually transmitted infections

TID	Tobacco Industry Denormalization
UNAIDS	United Nations Programme on HIV/AIDS
UNFPA	United Nations Population Fund
UNODC	United Nations Office on Drugs and Crime
WHO	World Health Organization

Introduction

Damien de Walque

Behaviors that pose risks to the health of individuals as well as to the general public are highly prevalent in both high-income and low-income countries. While many developing countries correctly consider the HIV/AIDS (human immunodeficiency virus/acquired immune deficiency syndrome) epidemic to be a key challenge, these countries perceive other risks only as emerging threats, in part because some of the risky behaviors may be associated with richer countries. This book reviews the evidence on these behaviors in developing countries. In particular, it investigates the determinants of such behaviors, summarizes their consequences, and reviews policy options available to governments to discourage them.

While many other behaviors—such as reckless driving or avoiding treatment for an infectious disease—pose substantial health risks to individuals and the public, this book focuses on behaviors that can have strong effects on the health of individuals, for which the existing literature is substantial, and for which the level of evidence is relatively high: using illicit drugs, smoking, consuming excessive amounts of alcohol, overeating, and engaging in risky sex.

Individual choices are an important part of the risky behaviors we examine. But how are those choices formed? Why do people engage in risky behaviors? Many different explanations have been proposed by specialists in the disciplines of psychology, sociology, economics, and public health. Risky behaviors have many characteristics and are multifaceted. But one trait that is common to them is the disconnect between the pleasure or satisfaction they provide and the consequences they entail. This disconnect is a function of both delay and uncertainty. If smoking killed quickly, few people would choose to light a cigarette. But there is usually a long lag between the enjoyment of the "guilty pleasure" and the negative health consequences. Moreover, these health behaviors are considered to be "risky" because the outcomes are not always certain. Not all smokers die from lung cancer, not all heavy drinkers suffer from liver cirrhosis, and not everyone who has multiple sexual partners without using condoms becomes HIV-positive.

Another characteristic of risky behaviors is that they rarely occur in isolation. Peer pressure, parental influences, networks, and social norms often play important roles in the choices to initiate, continue, or quit those behaviors. Even if individuals might be the first to suffer, the consequences of risky behaviors are rarely limited to those engaging in them. In certain cases, the link is direct: drug consumption, smoking, alcohol use, poor diet, and HIV and sexually transmitted infections (STIs) among mothers have detrimental impacts on their fetuses; second-hand smoking is a serious health hazard to others; and unprotected sex and needle-sharing lead to the spread of HIV and other STIs. In other cases, the link is less direct but not necessarily less real: the long-term health consequences of many of these behaviors are costly and could stretch households' finances and exacerbate poverty. Finally, these risky behaviors have consequences for society as a whole, since they often trigger significant public health expenditures and lead to declines in aggregate productivity through premature mortality and morbidity.

"Risk-taking" by individuals is determined by their valuation of health, their knowledge of the consequences of such behaviors, and the actions of others. One possible starting point is that individuals will make trade-offs between the benefits of risky and unhealthy behaviors—such as immediate pleasure or the satisfaction of addiction—and the costs of such behaviors—such as the market price of alcohol, drugs, tobacco, and unhealthy foods—and the potentially harmful consequences for their health and life expectancy (Cawley and Ruhm 2012; Grossman 1972, 2000).

While this concept of a trade-off is a useful starting point, this idea might appear difficult to reconcile with what we observe about those behaviors. Are people really making conscious trade-offs, especially once they are under the influence of substances that might cloud their judgment? Aren't some of these products creating addictions that are powerful and cannot be overcome by individuals exerting conscious choices? Are people well-informed about the health risks associated with those risky behaviors? Even if well-informed, are all people able to make adequate trade-offs between immediate pleasure and long-term risks? Isn't the very fact that many people engage in behaviors they know to be harmful evidence of the contrary? And to what extent are those people making those choices as isolated individuals, or as people influenced by their peers, their social networks, or social norms?

Given that these behaviors might be the results of a trade-off between immediate pleasure and long-term and uncertain negative health consequences, and since they may have consequences for others and society, it might be useful to adopt an economics lens to investigate the determinants and implications of risky behaviors. Further, interventions to reduce those risky behaviors, in addition to the direct regulation and the dissemination of information about the attendant risks, often include economic mechanisms such as taxes, subsidies, or conditional cash transfers.

Although the economic perspective is useful, it has its limitations. Insights from other disciplines such as psychology, sociology, or biology are also important. In order to better understand what motivates those behaviors and to consider different policy options for prevention, this book integrates recent advances in behavioral economics (DellaVigna 2009) and other disciplines that deal with such issues as cognitive limitations, addiction, information constraints, time-inconsistent preferences, and peer effects.

This volume summarizes the existing evidence from a broad range of sources at a time when the World Bank portfolio addressing risky behaviors for health is growing, but it does not explicitly serve as an overview of World Bank projects. It does, however, build on a rich body of work done in many regions.[1] The book has an explicit focus on low- and middle-income countries.[2] It attempts to be as comprehensive as possible in its synthesis of evidence, although it will not perform a meta-analysis or a systematic literature review. It includes studies from more developed countries, either because they are seminal contributions or recent systematic reviews, or because the evidence from developing countries is scant. When data and research gaps are such that the authors had to refer to evidence from high-income countries, the findings do not necessarily or automatically apply to the developing world. Finally, this book focuses on individual behaviors rather than on societal, cultural, or government behaviors or decisions, although the spillover effects, externalities, and peer effects are explicitly covered.

Different levels of evidence can be found. Causality is difficult to establish, but it is important to assess. The authors attempt to analyze the strength of the evidence presented in the surveyed studies, and they clearly distinguish between correlation and causation. Even if causality is important, correlations can be useful, especially when looking at determinants of risky behaviors, as they might help target interventions. However, when looking at studies evaluating the impact of interventions designed to prevent unhealthy behaviors, causal inference is key.

The opening chapter in this volume, by Damien de Walque and Sébastien Piguet, presents a rapid overview, illustrated by tables, figures, and maps, of the global prevalence and distribution of the risky behaviors that are the focus of this book. This epidemiological overview highlights emerging threats for public health and, to the extent that data are available, documents trends. Several of the risky behaviors traditionally associated with developed countries, such as smoking and obesity, have in recent decades become substantial threats to public health in the developing world as well.

The second chapter, by Mattias Lundberg and Gil Shapira, covers the determinants of health-related risky behaviors in the developing world. Individuals' perceptions of the benefits and eventual costs associated with these behaviors, as well as the manner in which they consider the trade-off between these benefits and costs, depend on many factors. These are individual factors such as socioeconomic background and subjective perceptions, as well as characteristics of the environment in which these decisions are being made, such as prices and social norms. The chapter explores how these factors can explain variations in such behaviors, both within populations as well as over time. Understanding the determinants of risky behaviors is crucial for designing effective policies. While some of these determinants can be directly changed by policy makers, others will entail individuals' responses to these policy changes. Furthermore, the association between different characteristics and risk-taking can guide better targeting of different policy interventions. Although the chapter starts from an economic point of view, it discusses how engagement in risky behaviors and response to policy changes are conditioned by psychological, social, and biological factors.

Chapter 3, by Alaka Holla, explores the consequences of risky behaviors, focusing on their direct impact on the individual engaging in them; the spillovers to peers in their immediate environment, such as family members or coworkers; and the costs that society must bear. These spillovers to peers and society are what economists call externalities—consequences of an activity experienced by third parties who cannot be compensated or charged for the costs or benefits they experience, thereby making it difficult for individuals to take these into account when deciding to engage in the activity. Smoking, for example, generates secondhand smoke that adversely affects the health of those exposed; obesity can lead to chronic conditions whose financial cost is often at least partially borne by the health system. In developing countries, the chronic diseases that often result from the risky behaviors examined may strike at younger ages than in wealthier countries, lengthening the periods of elevated health expenditures and compounding the productivity losses associated with the increases in morbidity. The review of findings from across the world reveals such large impacts that existing or emerging markets for insurance may not be able to handle the costs. The presence of large externalities to peers and society more generally clearly suggests that public intervention can improve overall welfare.

Chapters 4 and 5 discuss interventions to reduce the prevalence of risky behaviors. Chapter 4, by Aakanksha Pande, examines the effect of information, education, and communication (IEC) campaigns, as well as prohibition and regulation, while chapter 5 considers economic interventions based on incentives and price mechanisms. Given the public health consequences of risky behaviors, interventions have been developed to discourage them. Interventions based on information provision and legislation can be subdivided into *demand-side* interventions that target users (for example, education) and *supply-side* interventions that target producers (for example, regulation). Prohibition spans this by affecting both demand- and supply-side factors. This chapter summarizes the effectiveness of both categories of interventions.

Supply-side interventions primarily target regulation. This includes instituting a minimum legal drinking age and restricting the sale of alcohol and tobacco to minors; regulating the fatty content in foods and the sale of calorific beverages; imposing advertising bans on certain alcohol and tobacco products; and legalizing sex workers. Demand-side interventions focus on educating the consumer on the negative consequences of risky behaviors. These include providing graphic health warnings on cigarette packets; labeling the caloric value of foods; and offering information campaigns, counseling, and testing of those engaging in risky sex. Other demand-side interventions include providing users with physical tools to encourage safer behavior, for example, through needle exchange programs for drug users. Prohibition, a more extreme form of regulation, affects both users and producers. Most countries enforce prohibition of the use and sale of narcotics; prohibition of the use of alcohol has existed at different times. After the World Health Organization's promulgation in 2003 of the Framework Convention on Tobacco Control, prohibition of smoking in public places has been a widely enforced provision in the 174 ratifying countries.

The findings show that information and regulation interventions can be successful in changing risky behaviors. Evidence from both developed and developing countries suggests that legislation to change risky behaviors tends to be effective, especially if enforcement mechanisms are strong. In general, information and education campaigns have been effective in informing consumers about the risks associated with certain behaviors. But translating that knowledge into concrete changes in behavior seems to be harder to achieve. Across risky behaviors, certain enabling conditions emerge that make it more likely for an intervention to be effective. These conditions involve the design, targeting, or implementation of the intervention. Even if an intervention is effective, the duration of the effect varies and is a function of the length and intensity with which the intervention was delivered. Once the intervention is removed, there can be a "bounce back" effect to levels similar to those before the intervention was introduced.

An important lesson that emerges from this review is that even when interventions are effective, externalities often emerge that need to be considered. This is especially the case when a substance is banned, since substitution effects tend to occur. Before implementing a policy, policy makers need to think through all the potential effects that can result if it is effective and then try and preempt the negative consequences to the extent possible. At the very least, negative externalities should be assumed and included in the cost-benefit calculus before deciding to implement an intervention.

Complementing chapter 4, chapter 5, by Damien de Walque, reviews the use of economic mechanisms such as taxes (for example, on alcohol and smoking), subsidies (for example, on condoms), and conditional and unconditional cash transfers (for example, for prevention of HIV/STI and teenage pregnancy) as interventions to reduce risky behaviors. Taxes have been used widely in the developed world as a mechanism to reduce risky behaviors, such as alcohol and smoking, by increasing the price to consumers. Several developing countries are considering the introduction or increase of taxes on those products. Tax policies have been shown to be effective as instruments to prevent smoking and alcohol consumption, but so far they have been less effective for reducing the use of unhealthy food. Most of the evidence comes from developed countries, but an emerging literature from developing countries points in the same direction. Taxing unhealthy behaviors is an attractive policy option, since it also increases government revenue, even if it might encounter political opposition. Substitution across products and subcategories of products is a key issue to keep in mind when devising tax policies.

Subsidies have also been used, perhaps less frequently, to encourage safer behaviors. Examples include free or subsidized condoms or family planning. Beyond pure price interventions, incentives are also proposed as a mechanism to discourage risky behaviors or encourage safe behaviors. Demand-side interventions using financial incentives such as conditional cash transfers (CCTs) have been experimented with to incentivize safe sex, reduce the prevalence of STIs, and encourage weight loss. Similar to CCTs, contingency management relies on the mechanism of conditionality to elicit behaviors that are viewed to be in the long-term interests of individuals or society, and to discourage those behaviors that may be ultimately detrimental to individuals' health and well-being and that may not be easily perceived in the short term. Contingency management applications span many areas of risky behaviors, including abusing illicit substances, smoking, and overeating, but in general they have mainly been implemented and tested in developed countries. Finally, commitment devices in which participants commit their own funds or savings and get them back only if they satisfy conditions, such as not smoking or losing weight, have recently been experimented. The commitment mechanism explicitly recognizes the bounded rationality of individuals engaging in risky behaviors. Those experiments should be further encouraged, but they should also try to systematically test the existence of long-term or sustained impacts, since those are the most relevant for public health.

Notes

1. See, among others, Bonilla-Chacín and Marcano Vásquez (2012); Marquez (2005); Shrimpton and Rokx (forthcoming); and Wang, Marquez, and Langenbrunner (2011).
2. For operational and analytical purposes, the World Bank's main criterion for classifying economies is gross national income (GNI) per capita. Economies are divided according to 2011 GNI per capita, calculated using the World Bank Atlas method. The groups are low-income, US$1,025 or less; lower-middle-income, US$1,026 to $4,035; upper-middle-income, US$4,036 to $12,475; and high-income, US$12,476 or more.

References

Bonilla-Chacín, María E., and Luis T. Marcano Vásquez. 2012. "Promoting Healthy Living in Latin America and the Caribbean: Multi-Sectoral Approaches to Preventing Noncommunicable Diseases." Health, Nutrition, and Population Discussion Paper 71848, World Bank, Washington, DC.

Cawley, John, and Christopher J. Ruhm. 2012. "The Economics of Risky Health Behaviors." In *Handbook of Health Economics*, vol. 2, edited by Pedro Pita Barros, Tom McGuire, and Mark Pauly, 95–199. New York: Elsevier.

DellaVigna, Stefano. 2009. "Psychology and Economics: Evidence from the Field." *Journal of Economic Literature* 47 (2): 315–72.

Grossman, Michael. 1972. "On the Concept of Health Capital and the Demand for Health." *Journal of Political Economy* 80 (2): 223–49.

———. 2000. "The Human Capital Model." In *Handbook of Health Economics*, vol. 1A, edited by Anthony J. Culyer and Joseph P. Newhouse, 347–408. New York: Elsevier.

Marquez, Patricio V. 2005. *Dying Too Young: Addressing Premature Mortality and Ill Health Due to Non-communicable Diseases and Injuries in the Russian Federation*. Washington, DC: World Bank.

Shrimpton, Roger, and Claudia Rokx. Forthcoming. "The Double Burden of Malnutrition: A Review of Global Evidence." Health, Nutrition, and Population Discussion Paper, World Bank, Washington, DC.

Wang Shiyon, Patricio V. Marquez, and John Langenbrunner. 2011. "Toward a Healthy and Harmonious Life in China: Stemming the Rising Tide of Non-communicable Diseases." Report 62318-CN, Human Development Unit, East Asia and Pacific Region, World Bank, Washington, DC.

1

Overview of the Prevalence and Trends of Risky Behaviors in the Developing World

Damien de Walque and Sébastien Piguet

Introduction

This chapter presents an overview of the prevalence of risky behaviors across the world and across time, when data on trends are available. Although the focus is on risky behaviors, their consequences also are discussed. Illegal drug use ultimately leads to overdoses and HIV infection, smoking causes lung cancer, alcohol abuse leads to cirrhosis of the liver, unhealthy diets and lack of exercise lead to obesity, and risky sex increases the likelihood of HIV and other sexually transmitted infections and teenage pregnancies.

Data Collection Challenges

Data collection about risky behaviors is challenging, in part because of self-reporting biases. Measuring trends and prevalence and comparing them across countries are problematic because of the difficulties finding precise information on both the behaviors and their consequences. Smoking and alcohol consumption are relatively easy to measure through surveys; however, unhealthy diets, lack of exercise, and risky sex are more complex behaviors that are more difficult to capture and summarize in a few survey questions. However, independently of whether they are complex, it is important to stress that in surveys all of these behaviors are self-reported, which might result in biases (Brener, Billy, and Grady 2003). Social desirability bias, in particular, might be an important issue, since many of those behaviors are frowned upon by society and individuals might be reluctant to acknowledge them in a survey.

These behaviors are also more context-specific: what constitutes a healthy diet varies across countries and also depends on age, occupation, and level of activity. Casual sex with a one-night encounter might be very risky in a country in which HIV prevalence among adults is above 15 percent, but less so when that prevalence is below 1 percent. For those reasons and because comparable data across countries and over time are not always available, the sections on illegal drugs, tobacco, and alcohol tend to focus on the measure of the behaviors themselves, providing information about consequences when available, while the sections on unhealthy diet and risky sex tend to focus on the measurable consequences of those behaviors, that is, obesity, HIV infection, and teenage pregnancy.

Illicit Drug Use

The United Nations Office on Drugs and Crime (UNODC 2012) estimates that globally between 153 and 300 million people, or 3.4 percent to 6.6 percent of the population ages 15–64, used illicit substances at least once in 2010. About half are current drug users, who have used illicit drugs at least once during the past month prior to the survey. The UNODC classifies illicit drug use into six main categories:

- Cannabis, with a global prevalence of 2.6 to 5.0 percent in 2010
- Opioids (mainly heroin, morphine, and nonmedical use of prescription opioids) with a global prevalence of 0.6 to 0.8 percent
- Opiates (a subset of opioids, including opium and heroin) with a global prevalence of 0.3 to 0.5 percent
- Cocaine, with a global prevalence of 0.3 to 0.4 percent
- Amphetamine-type stimulants (ATS), with the exception of ecstasy, with a global prevalence of 0.3 percent to 1.2 percent
- Ecstasy, with a global prevalence from 0.2 percent to 0.6 percent.

Prevalence

The prevalence of drug use among adults ages 15–64 is generally higher in the developed world (from 14.7 percent to15.1 percent in North America, 12.3 percent to 20.1 percent in Oceania, and 6.4 percent to 6.8 percent in Europe) than in developing regions (3.8 percent to 12.5 percent in Africa, 3.2 percent to 4.2 percent in Latin America and the Caribbean, and 1.4 percent to 4.6 percent in Asia) (UNODC 2012).

The UNODC (2012), however, warns about considerable challenges in the reporting of data on illicit drug use. The main challenges are the availability and reporting of data on different aspects of illicit drug demand and supply by each country. The paucity is particularly acute in Africa and parts of Asia, where data on the prevalence and trends remain vague at best.

Table 1.1 reports the estimated usage for the six drug groups by continent and subregions. Even though cannabis use is the most widespread in every world region, it is not necessarily the drug used by problem users. The UNODC (2012) defines a problem user as a user with drug dependence and/or drug-use disorders. Opioids are the drugs most likely to be problem drugs in Asia (59 percent of all problem drugs) and in Eastern and Southeastern Europe (76 percent), while cocaine (50 percent) followed by cannabis are

Table 1.1 Annual Prevalence of Drug Use by World Region

Region	Cannabis	Opioids	Opiates	Cocaine	ATS	Ecstasy
Africa	7.80	0.40	0.40	0.50	0.80	0.20
East Africa	4.20	0.40	0.40	0	0	0
North Africa	5.70	0.30	0.30	0.03	0	0
Southern Africa	5.40	0.40	0.30	0.80	0.70	0.40
West and Central Africa	12.40	0.40	0.40	0.70	0	0
Americas	6.60	2.10	0.20	1.20	0.90	0.50
Caribbean	2.80	0.40	0.30	0.70	0.80	0.30
Central America	2.40	0.50	0.10	0.50	1.30	0.10
North America	10.80	4.00	0.40	1.60	1.30	0.90
South America	2.50	0.30	0.04	0.70	0.50	0.20
Asia	1.90	0.40	0.40	0.05	0.70	0.40
Central Asia	3.90	0.90	0.80	0	0	0
East and Southeast Asia	0.60	0.30	0.30	0.03	0.60	0.20
Near and Middle East	3.10	1.10	1.00	0.03	0.20	0
South Asia	3.60	0.30	0.30	0	0	0
Europe	5.20	0.70	0.50	0.80	0.50	0.70
Eastern and Southeastern Europe	2.70	1.20	0.80	0.20	0.30	0.60
Western and Central Europe	6.90	0.40	0.30	1.30	0.60	0.80
Oceania	10.90	3.00	0.20	1.50	2.10	2.90

Source: UNODC 2011.

Note: ATS = amphetamine-type stimulants.

the most problematic drugs in Latin America and the Caribbean, and cannabis (64 percent) is the main problem drug in Africa (UNODC 2011).

Because the UNODC (2011) data only report estimates for each drug group separately, it is difficult to obtain statistics about drug use in general, such as calculating the percentage of individuals who use any type of drug. Indeed, adding the numbers for each drug group would run the risk of double-counting since individuals might be using different types of drugs concurrently. For this reason, we cannot include, like we do for other countries, a map illustrating the worldwide distribution of drug use and a table with the countries with the highest prevalence. The UNODC (2011, 2012) does not include extensive data disaggregated by gender, but it notes in general that illicit drug use among males greatly exceeds that among females. A notable exception, however, is the use of tranquilizers and sedatives, which is higher among females (UNODC 2012).

Mortality

Worldwide estimates indicate that from 99,000 to 253,000 adults die each year from drug-related causes, corresponding to a mortality rate per million of 22 to 55.9. Using and aggregating data reported by each country, UNODC (2012) estimates the number of drug-related deaths and mortality rates per million population ages 15 to 64. The definitions and methods of recording drug-related deaths vary by country but comprise some or all of the following: unintentional overdose; suicide; HIV and AIDS acquired through the sharing of contaminated drug paraphernalia; and trauma, such as motor vehicle accidents caused by driving under the influence of illicit drugs. Mortality from drug use is higher in the developed world (147.3 per million in North America, 123.0 in Oceania, and 35.8 in Europe) than in the developing world (22.9 to 73.5 in Africa, 12.2 to 31.1 in Latin America and the Caribbean, and 5.4 to 48.6 in Asia).

While drug use might appear to be a "rich country" problem, the prevalence of drug use and drug-related deaths is not negligible in the developing world and should be given full consideration. Furthermore, even though this is beyond the scope of this chapter, it is worth noting that many drugs are made from products grown in the developing world (for example, coca and opium); accordingly, the consumption and illegal trade of drugs in developed countries affects the economy and the governance of many developing countries.

Stability of Drug Use

During the last decade, the worldwide prevalence of drug use—the proportion of drug users among the population ages 15–64—remained almost unchanged at approximately 5 percent (UNODC 2011). It is difficult to find reliable data to look at trends before the late 1990s and to disaggregate the trends by regions.

Smoking

Close to 20 percent of the world's adult population smokes cigarettes[1] (Eriksen, Mackay, and Ross 2012). Global cigarette consumption increased over 100 times from 1900 to 2000, going from 50 billion cigarettes to 5,711 billion in 2000 and 5,884 billion in 2009. Over the same period, the world's population grew from 1.7 billion in 1900, to 6 billion in 2000, and 7 billion in 2012 (United States Census Bureau 2013). These numbers imply that global consumption per year and per capita increased from 29 to 952 between 1900 and 2000. The vast majority of the world's smokers live in low- and middle-income countries. In 2009, China consumed more than 38 percent of the world's cigarettes (2,265 billion). The next four countries in cigarette consumption were the Russian Federation, the United States, Indonesia, and Japan (with 390, 316, 261, and 234 billion, respectively).

Maps 1.1 and 1.2 illustrate the percentage of male and female adults who were current cigarette smokers in 2010 or the latest available date. As for much of the information in this section, the information comes from

Map 1.1   Males Who Smoke Cigarettes, 2010 or latest available data

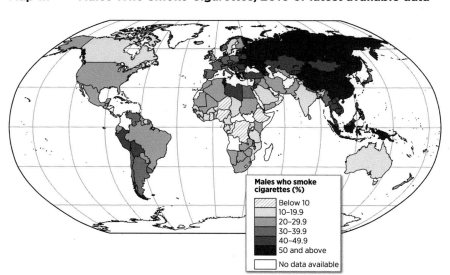

Males who smoke cigarettes (%)

- Below 10
- 10–19.9
- 20–29.9
- 30–39.9
- 40–49.9
- 50 and above
- No data available

Source: Eriksen, Mackay, and Ross 2012.

Map 1.2 Females Who Smoke Cigarettes, 2010 or latest available data

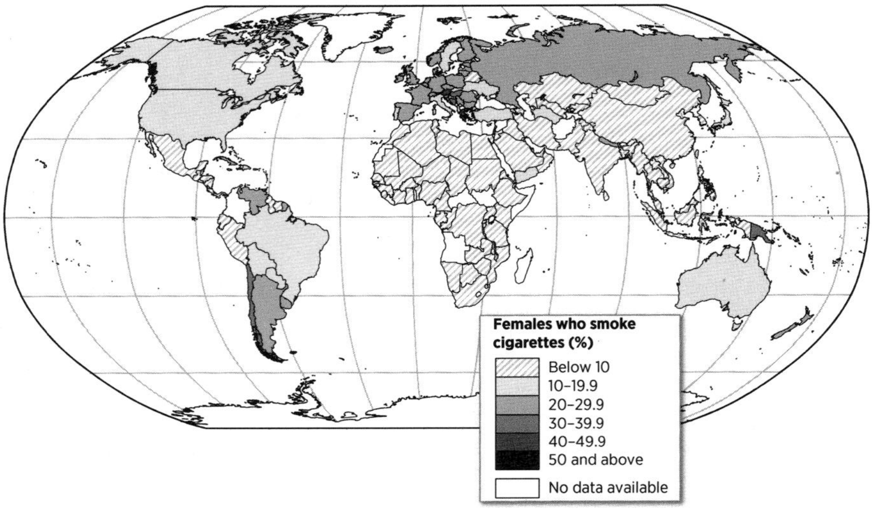

Source: Eriksen, Mackay, and Ross 2012.

Eriksen, Mackay, and Ross (2012)[2] and is compiled from self-reported data. Table 1.2 includes the prevalence of smoking among males in the 15 countries with highest measures.[3]

Generally, cigarette smoking is highest in East Asia, the former Soviet Union, Eastern Europe, a few countries in the Middle East (Libya and Tunisia), and Latin America and the Caribbean (Bolivia, Peru, and Cuba). Smoking among adult males is lowest (below 10 percent) in Oman and a few African countries.

In most countries, women are less likely to smoke; indeed, in many countries, they are only one-tenth as likely to smoke as men. Those countries include China, India, and Indonesia, as well as many other countries in East and South Asia, Africa, and the Middle East. Table 1.3 includes the 15 countries with the highest percentage of female smokers. The prevalence of female cigarette smoking is from 20 to 40 percent in most European countries and the Pacific Islands, Nepal, Argentina, Chile, Cuba, and República Bolivariana de Venezuela.

Mortality

In 2011, tobacco use killed close to 6 million people, with nearly 80 percent of these deaths in developing countries (Eriksen, Mackay, and Ross 2012).

Table 1.2 Countries with Highest Percentage of Male Smokers

Country	Prevalence
Kiribati	71.0
Greece	63.0
Albania	60.1
Russian Federation	58.6
Samoa	58.0
Papua New Guinea	57.7
Indonesia	57.2
Georgia	56.6
Tunisia	52.7
Armenia	50.9
Tuvalu	50.8
China	50.4
Latvia	50.1
Ukraine	50.0
Lithuania	49.9
Korea, Rep.	49.3

Source: Eriksen, Mackay, and Ross 2012.

While maps 1.1 and 1.2 and the prevalence by country paint a contrasting picture of developed and developing countries, the trends reveal another dynamic. In many developed countries, smoking prevalence peaked in the 1960s or early 1970s, a few years after the information about the health dangers of tobacco became widespread. In 1960, smoking prevalence among males was 81 percent in Japan, 61 percent in the United Kingdom, and 52 percent in the United States. Fifty years later in 2010, those numbers were 38 percent in Japan, and 22 percent in the United Kingdom and the United States. Trends for females were similar, even though the starting point was lower; between 1960 and 2010, smoking prevalence declined from 13 to 11 percent in Japan, from 42 to 21 percent in the United Kingdom, and from 34 to 17 percent in the United States (Eriksen, Mackay, and Ross 2012).

Increasing Prevalence in Developing Countries

While smoking prevalence is decreasing in developed countries, it is increasing in many developing countries. Data constraints make

Table 1.3   Countries with Highest Percentage of Female Smokers

Country	Prevalence
Nauru	50.0
Austria	45.1
Kiribati	42.9
Greece	41.4
Bosnia and Herzegovina	35.6
Hungary	33.5
Andorra	32.3
Cook Islands	31.2
Papua New Guinea	30.8
Lebanon	30.7
Luxembourg	30.4
Chile	30.2
Croatia	29.6
Cuba	29.4
Nepal	28.4

Source: Eriksen, Mackay, and Ross 2012.

ascertaining trends more difficult for developing countries.[4] In some middle-income countries like Brazil and Turkey, the prevalence has also been trending downward recently (INCA 2010; Ministry of Health [Turkey] 2010). However, using a weighted average of smoking prevalence, Eriksen, Mackay, and Ross (2012) describe four stages of a tobacco epidemic continuum over a century (figures 1.1 and 1.2).

- The first stage, the first 20 years, is characterized by rising smoking prevalence and low smoking-related mortality. The female tobacco epidemic in low-income countries with 3 percent prevalence can still be placed in this stage.
- The second stage, between years 20 and 50, is characterized by a sharp increase in smoking prevalence, but because of the lag between current smoking and deaths attributed to tobacco, mortality increases more moderately. Low- and middle-income countries are currently in this phase for males, with average smoking prevalence 21 percent for low-income countries and 34 percent for middle-income countries. With 5 percent smoking prevalence among females, the tobacco epidemic in middle-income countries is at the threshold between stage 1 and stage 2.

Figure 1.1   The Tobacco Continuum and the Four Stages of the Smoking Epidemic in Males

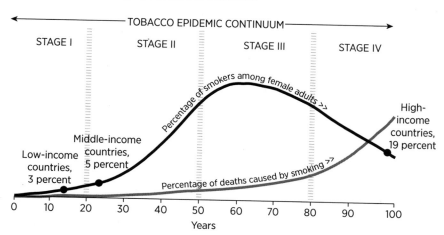

2010 smoking prevalence data overlaid on tobacco epidemic continuum

Source: Eriksen, Mackay, and Ross 2012.

Figure 1.2   The Tobacco Continuum and the Four Stages of the Smoking Epidemic in Females

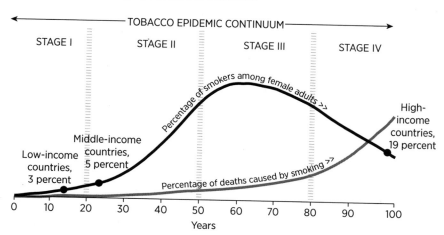

2010 smoking prevalence data overlaid on tobacco epidemic continuum

Source: Eriksen, Mackay, and Ross 2012.

- The third stage of the tobacco epidemic, between years 50 and 80, is characterized by a plateau and then a decrease in smoking prevalence, but with a sharp rise in tobacco-related mortality. Most high-income countries experienced this third stage from the 1960s to the 1990s.
- Most high-income countries are in the fourth stage of the tobacco continuum, from year 80 to year 100, with a continued decrease in smoking prevalence (30 percent among males and 19 percent among females) and the beginning of a decrease in mortality caused by smoking.

Alcohol Consumption

Map 1.3 illustrates the per capita consumption for adults in liters of pure alcohol and the geographical distribution. The data come from the Global Information System on Alcohol and Health (GISAH)[5] developed by the World Health Organization (WHO) (2011). It is important to acknowledge some data limitations due to "unrecorded consumption," such as home brewing, illegal production, travelers' imports, and consumption by residents outside the country.[6] Table 1.4 includes the countries with the highest consumption patterns.

Map 1.3   Total Adult Per Capita Consumption, in liters of pure alcohol, 2008 or latest available

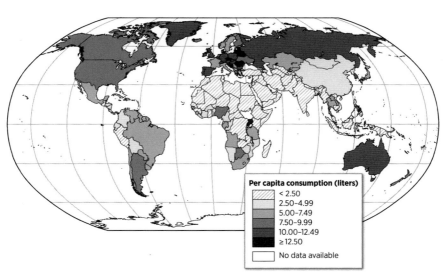

Source: World Health Organization (WHO) 2013.
Note: Adult = persons over age 15.

Table 1.4   Countries with Highest Per Capita Consumption of Alcohol, liters of pure alcohol

Country	Per capita consumption
Virgin Islands (U.S.)	23.4
British Virgin Islands	22.8
Moldova	20.6
Cayman Islands	20.5
Cook Islands	18.0
Aruba	17.3
Luxembourg	15.3
Netherlands Antilles	15.2
Czech Republic	15.0
Belarus	13.8
Bosnia and Herzegovina	13.5
Uganda	13.4
Latvia	13.2
Romania	12.7
Lithuania	12.6

Source: WHO 2011.

With the exception of small islands and Uganda, most of the locations are in Europe, including the Russian Federation and other countries from the former Soviet Union. Several countries in Asia, the Middle East and North Africa, and Sub-Saharan Africa—many with a predominant Muslim population—have the lowest levels (below 2.5 liters per year).

Map 1.4 illustrates the impact of alcohol consumption on adult mortality[7] across the world.

Excessive Consumption Unhealthy

Unlike drugs or tobacco for which even modest consumption is unhealthy, only excessive alcohol consumption constitutes an unhealthy behavior. It is less risky to drink, during a week, two glasses of alcohol every day with a meal than to drink the same number of drinks (14) on Friday and Saturday evenings. The Global Status Report on Alcohol and Health (WHO 2011) developed the patterns of drinking score (PDS), which reflects *how* people drink instead of *how much* they drink.[8] Strongly associated with the alcohol-attributable burden of disease of a country, the PDS is measured on a scale

Map 1.4   Alcohol-Attributable Deaths as a Percentage of Total Deaths, 2004

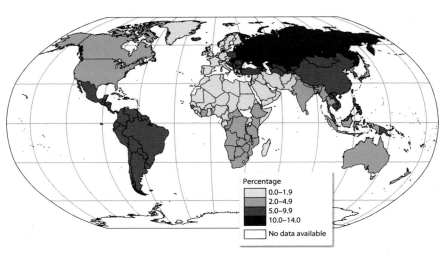

Percentage
- 0.0–1.9
- 2.0–4.9
- 5.0–9.9
- 10.0–14.0
- No data available

Source: WHO 2011.

from 1 (least risky pattern of drinking) to 5 (most risky pattern of drinking). It is based on a set of drinking attributes, which include the usual quantity of alcohol consumed per occasion, festive drinking, the proportion of drinking events that lead to drunkenness, the proportion of drinkers that drink daily or nearly daily, drinking with meals, and drinking in public places. Map 1.5 displays the distribution of the PDS across the globe, and table 1.5 shows the countries with the most risky pattern of drinking (5 and 4), which is consistent with the patterns described in map 1.4 illustrating alcohol-related mortality.

Most of South America, and many countries in Africa and Southeast Asia, are in an intermediate position, while several countries in Western and Southern Europe have the least risky drinking patterns, despite a fairly high level of per capita consumption. Trends of alcohol consumption between 1990 and 2005, including the recorded adult per capita consumption, have been fairly stable both globally and within regions (WHO 2011).

Gender Differences

Few of the estimates on alcohol consumption published by the WHO (2011) are disaggregated by gender. The percentage of students who drank at least one drink containing alcohol on one or more of the past 30 days

Map 1.5   Patterns of Drinking Score by Country, 2005

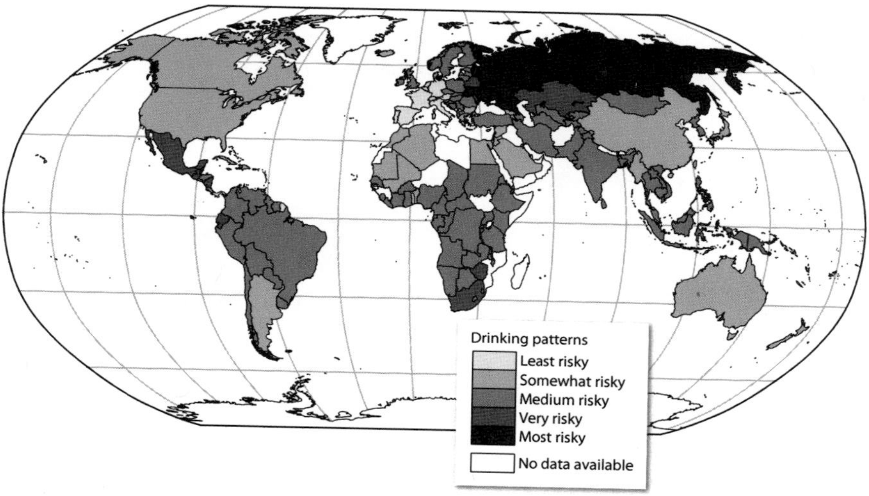

Drinking patterns
- Least risky
- Somewhat risky
- Medium risky
- Very risky
- Most risky
- No data available

Source: WHO 2013.

Table 1.5   Countries with Highest Patterns of Drinking Score (PDS)

Country	PDS
Russian Federation	5
Ukraine	5
Belarus	4
Belize	4
Ecuador	4
Guatemala	4
Kazakhstan	4
Mexico	4
Moldova	4
Nicaragua	4
South Africa	4
Zimbabwe	4

Source: WHO 2011.

was only slightly higher among males than among females in most countries. However, women are more likely to completely abstain from alcohol, and men are usually much more likely to engage in heavy-drinking episodes, defined as drinking at least 60 grams or more of pure alcohol on at least one occasion in the past seven days.

Overweight and Obesity

Dietary risks are complex and difficult to measure; accordingly, to have comparable data across countries and over time, we focus on the prevalence and trends of their more easily observable consequences—obesity and overweight among individuals over age 15—based on recent WHO data. Adults are considered *overweight* if their body mass index (BMI)— their weight in kilograms divided by their height in meters squared (kg/m^2)—is equal to or greater than 25, and *obese* if their BMI is equal to or greater than 30. There is some debate about these thresholds. First, for men, overweight might indicate muscularity rather than fatness. Indeed, BMI is a useful but imperfect measure because it does not actually measure fat, and it ignores body composition by failing to distinguish between kilograms of muscle and kilograms of fat (Burkhauser and Cawley 2008). Also, the threshold could be lower in regions where people generally have lower muscle mass, such as in East Asia. Despite these caveats, being overweight, especially being obese, puts individuals at risk for many health problems, such as coronary heart disease, high blood pressure, type 2 diabetes, gallstones, and respiratory problems. We show the distribution and trends of being overweight or obese, with the understanding that obesity denotes a much higher risk.

Obesity in the Developing World

While the highest proportion of overweight and obese individuals is in the developed world, several regions or countries from the developing world, especially in the Middle East and Latin America and the Caribbean, are starting to experience high rates of overweight. Map 1.6 illustrates the distribution of overweight males (BMI > 25); map 1.7 displays the same geographical distribution of overweight females. Geographical patterns are similar for males and females, but the prevalence of overweight is generally higher among females, except in Australia and most of North America and Europe. Maps 1.8 and 1.9 depict the distribution of obesity (BMI > 30 kg/m^2). In most countries, less than 20 percent of males are obese, but a few countries have rates between 20 and 35 percent. Tables 1.6 and 1.7 list the 15 countries with the highest prevalence of obesity among males and

Map 1.6   Male Overweight (BMI > 25) Prevalence by Country, 2008

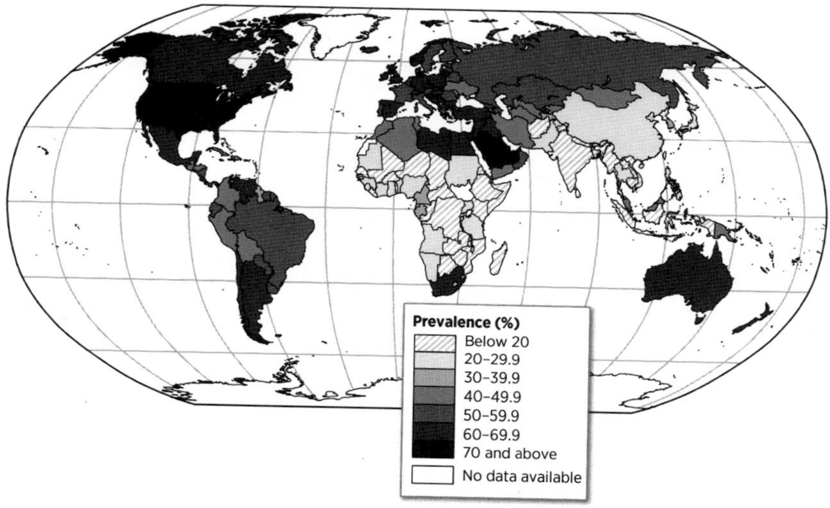

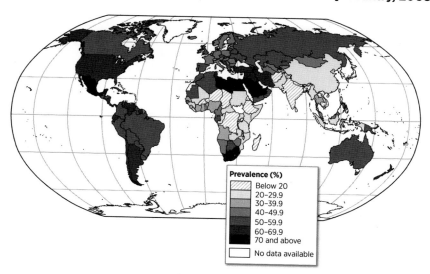

Source: WHO 2011.
Note: Data are for people ages 20 years and older.

Map 1.7   Female Overweight (BMI > 25) Prevalence by Country, 2008

Source: WHO 2011.
Note: Data are for people ages 20 years and older.

Map 1.8   **Male Obesity (BMI > 30) Prevalence by Country, 2008**

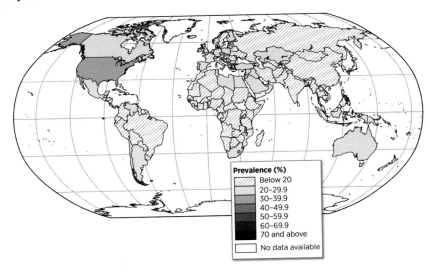

Source: WHO 2013.
Note: Data are for people ages 20 years and older.

Map 1.9   **Female Obesity (BMI > 30) Prevalence by Country, 2008**

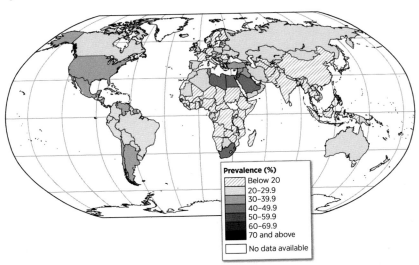

Source: WHO 2013.
Note: Data are for people ages 20 years and older.

Table 1.6   Countries with Highest Percentage of Obese Males, 2008

Country	Prevalence
Nauru	67.5
Cook Islands	59.7
Tonga	49.1
Samoa	45.3
Palau	44.9
Marshall Islands	38.8
Kiribati	37.7
Kuwait	37.2
St. Kitts and Nevis	32.0
Micronesia, Fed. Sts.	30.9
Qatar	30.8
Czech Republic	30.5
United Arab Emirates	30.2
United States	30.2
Saudi Arabia	29.5

Source: WHO 2013.

females, respectively. Obesity is more prevalent among women in Europe, Oceania, the Middle East and North Africa, and North and South America, with prevalence rates between 20 and 35 percent, and between 25 and 50 percent in several countries as illustrated in map 1.9. Rates of overweight and obesity are also very high for both males and females in some islands in the Pacific.

Dietary Risks

Dietary risks—the health risks associated with an unbalanced diet—have become the leading factor contributing to the global burden of disease. Data on trends of overweight, obesity, and dietary risks across the world are limited, especially from developing countries. The Institute for Health Metrics and Evaluation (2013) produces estimates of the ranking of risks contributing to the global burden of disease. For the developing world as a whole in 1990, childhood underweight (defined as weight 2 standard deviations below the mean weight for age of the National Center for Health Statistics and the WHO reference population) was the leading factor, whereas dietary risks—health risks due

Table 1.7   Countries with Highest Percentage of Obese Females, 2008

Country	Prevalence
Nauru	74.7
Tonga	70.3
Cook Islands	68.5
Samoa	66.7
Palau	56.3
Marshall Islands	53.9
Kiribati	53.6
Micronesia, Fed. Sts.	53.4
Kuwait	52.4
St. Kitts and Nevis	49.4
Egypt, Arab Rep.	46.3
Belize	45.4
Barbados	44.2
Saudi Arabia	43.5
United Arab Emirates	43.0

Source: WHO 2013.

to unbalanced diet composition—was third, and high BMI was 15th. By 2010, however, dietary risks were first, and childhood underweight was fifth, while a high body-mass index was 10 and physical inactivity 12, illustrating the rise of dietary risks, physical inactivity, and overweight or obesity as risk factors for health in the developing world. By 2010, dietary risks were estimated to be the main contributing risk to the burden of disease in East Asia, South Asia, Southeast Asia, Latin America and the Caribbean, and the Middle East and North Africa. Bonilla-Chacín (2012) illustrates this in detail for Latin America and the Caribbean. It is only in Sub-Saharan Africa that childhood underweight remained the main contributing factor, but even there, dietary risks moved from position 11 to position 7 in the ranking of risk factors between 1990 and 2010.

Rising Rates of Overweight and Obesity in Developing Countries

Overweight and obesity are on the rise in developing countries and coexist with underweight. Figures 1.3 through 1.6 show trends in

Figure 1.3 **Trends in Overweight Males (BMI > 25) in Brazil, China, Mexico, and South Africa**

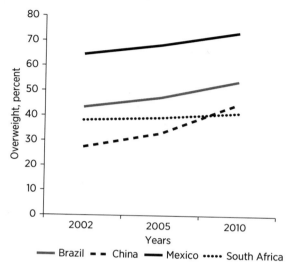

Source: WHO 2013.

Figure 1.4 **Trends in Obese Males (BMI > 30) in Brazil, China, Mexico, and South Africa**

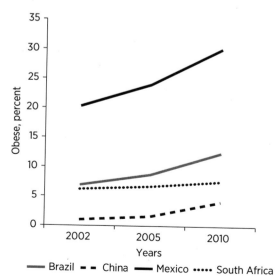

Source: WHO 2013.

Figure 1.5 **Trends in Overweight Females (BMI > 25) in Brazil, China, Mexico, and South Africa**

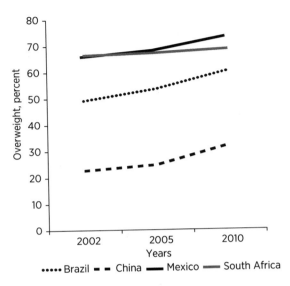

Source: WHO 2013.

Figure 1.6 **Trends in Obese Females (BMI > 30) in Brazil, China, Mexico, and South Africa**

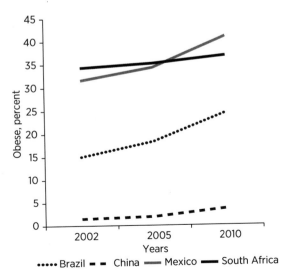

Source: WHO 2013.

overweight and obesity prevalence of males and females in Brazil, China, Mexico, and South Africa, using 2002, 2005, and 2010 data. These figures illustrate these increasing trends over a limited period of eight years for only four countries; however, these are large countries that are fairly representative of their region. A comparison over the years clearly indicates a general increase in the proportion of individuals who are either overweight or obese, for both genders. These trends indicate that the overweight and obesity epidemic is rapidly growing in many developing countries. Many of these countries might be in the middle of a "nutrition transition" (Popkin 2001), going relatively quickly from a situation in which a large percentage of the population is underweight or malnourished to a situation where a large percentage of the population is overweight or obese. We are now confronted with the paradox of the coexistence of both undernutrition and overnutrition in the same population across the life course, a paradox that has been labeled as the double burden of malnutrition. The concept recognizes that undernutrition early in the life course contributes to an increased propensity for overnutrition in adulthood (Shrimpton and Rokx 2013).

Risky Sex

Risky sex is a behavior that is difficult to measure in surveys, because sexual behaviors are particularly prone to self-reporting bias. In addition, a combination of behaviors is often needed for the sexual encounter to be risky, such as casual sex and the absence of condom use. Finally, the context is important: casual unprotected sex is much more risky when the HIV prevalence among the pool of partners is high. Risky sex can have many serious consequences, such as sexually transmitted diseases, including HIV/AIDS, and unwanted and teenage pregnancies. We highlight two consequences, HIV/AIDS and teenage pregnancies, to examine their global prevalence as proxies for the prevalence of risky sexual behavior.

HIV/AIDS

Globally, 34.0 million people were living with HIV at the end of 2011 (UNAIDS 2012). While risky sex is not the only behavior leading to HIV infection,[9] it remains the predominant transmission channel. HIV prevalence numbers are reported by UNAIDS based on reports sent by each country. In the high-prevalence countries, the HIV prevalence estimates are usually obtained from nationally representative surveys, such as

Demographic and Health Surveys. Compared to the majority of risky behaviors, HIV status is not self-reported but is the result of a serological test. However, in those surveys, HIV testing is recommended but not compulsory. Therefore, test refusals or absences during the test might still introduce some biases.

Sub-Saharan Africa

Sub-Saharan Africa has the larger share—69 percent—of all people living with HIV worldwide. An estimated 0.8 percent of adults ages 15–49 years worldwide are living with HIV, although the burden of the epidemic varies considerably among countries and regions. Map 1.10 illustrates this geographic variation. Sub-Saharan Africa is most severely affected, with nearly 1 in every 20 adults (4.9 percent) living with HIV. Within Sub-Saharan Africa, the southern cone of the continent—Botswana, Lesotho, South Africa, and Swaziland—is the most affected. Table 1.8 includes the 15 countries with the highest HIV prevalence among the adult population. We do not disaggregate the HIV prevalence data by gender; even though some differences in HIV prevalence by gender exist (in Sub-Saharan Africa, the region most

Map 1.10   Adult HIV Prevalence by Country, 2011

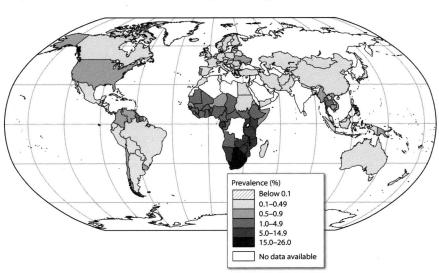

Source: World Bank 2013.

Table 1.8   Countries with Highest HIV Prevalence

Country	Prevalence
Swaziland	26.0
Botswana	23.4
Lesotho	23.3
South Africa	17.3
Zimbabwe	14.9
Namibia	13.4
Zambia	12.5
Mozambique	11.3
Malawi	10.0
Uganda	7.2
Kenya	6.2
Tanzania	5.8
Gabon	5.0
Equatorial Guinea	4.7
Cameroon	4.6

Source: World Bank 2013.

severely affected, women represent 58 percent of the people living with HIV), and even if the age profile of HIV infection varies substantially by gender, with women infected earlier, the overall picture in terms of geographical distribution of the HIV epidemic is similar for both genders.

The prevalence of HIV infection is nearly 25 times higher in Sub-Saharan Africa than in Asia. Nevertheless, almost 5 million people are living with HIV in South, Southeast, and East Asia combined. After Sub-Saharan Africa, the two regions most heavily affected are Latin America and the Caribbean, and Eastern Europe and Central Asia, where 1.0 percent of adults were living with HIV in 2011 (UNAIDS 2012).

Global decline in HIV

Worldwide, the rates of new infections and of mortality continue to fall. The number of adults and children acquiring HIV infection in 2011 was 2.5 million, 25 percent lower than in 2001 (UNAIDS 2012). The sharpest declines in the numbers of people acquiring HIV infection since 2001 have occurred in Latin America and the Caribbean (42 percent) and Sub-Saharan Africa (25 percent). In other parts of the world, HIV trends are cause for concern. Since 2001, the number of people newly infected in the Middle East and North Africa has increased by more than 35 percent (from 27,000 to 37,000). Evidence indicates that the incidence of HIV infection in Eastern Europe and Central Asia began increasing in the late 2000s after being relatively stable for several years.

The number of people dying from AIDS-related causes began to decline in the mid-2000s because of scaled-up antiretroviral therapy—a life-saving treatment that prolongs the lives of AIDS patients—and the steady decline in HIV incidence since the peak in 1997. In 2011, 1.7 million people died from AIDS-related causes worldwide, a 24 percent decline in AIDS-related mortality compared with 2005 (UNAIDS 2012).

Among generalized epidemic countries (HIV prevalence greater than 1 percent in the general population), country-reported HIV prevalence is consistently higher among sex workers, with a median of 23 percent, in the capital city than among the general population (UNAIDS 2012), and median country-reported HIV prevalence among sex workers in the capital cities remained stable between 2006 and 2011. Similarly, recent review of available data, which estimated the global HIV prevalence among female sex workers at 12 percent, found that female sex workers were 13.5 times more likely to be living with HIV than were other women (Kerrigan and others 2013; UNFPA, UNAIDS, and Asia Pacific Network of Sex Workers, forthcoming). HIV prevalence among female sex workers varied significantly by region, with the highest prevalence found in Sub-Saharan Africa, with a pooled prevalence of 36.9 percent (Kerrigan and others 2013).

Teenage Pregnancy

While pregnancy is not a risky behavior in itself, teenage pregnancies often have detrimental consequences. Pregnant teens are less likely to receive prenatal care, often seeking it only in the third trimester, if at all (UNICEF 2008). As a result of insufficient prenatal care and other reasons, the global incidence of premature births and low birth weight is higher among teenage mothers. Complications during pregnancy and delivery are the leading causes of death for girls ages 15 to 19 in developing countries, who are twice as likely to die in childbirth as women in their 20s. Teenage girls account for 14 percent of the estimated 20 million unsafe abortions performed each year, which result in some 68,000 deaths.

Teen pregnancy and childbearing are also associated with substantial social and economic costs through immediate and long-term impacts on teen parents and their children, such as school dropout rates for the girls, and lower educational achievement and poorer health outcomes for the children (Centers for Disease Control and Prevention 2013). However, these conclusions are debated; studies using miscarriages as natural experiments have estimated that teen births have no causal effect on education and labor market outcomes, since girls who become pregnant as teenagers are also more likely to have poor outcomes anyway (Hotz, Mullin, and Sanders 1997; Hotz, Williams McElroy, and Sanders 2005).

Fertility rates among women ages 15–19

Age-specific fertility rates for women ages 15–19 are highest in Sub-Saharan Africa. Map 1.11 illustrates the age-specific fertility rates (the number of births occurring during a year per 1,000 women classified by age group) for young women ages 15–19 for selected countries in which a Demographic and Health Survey was conducted between 2006 and 2011. The fertility rates (births divided by number of women ages 15 to 19) are expressed per 1,000 women and are for the period of 1 to 36 months preceding the survey. In all Sub-Saharan countries included, with the exception of Rwanda, the fertility rate was above 100.

Map 1.11   Age-Specific Fertility Rate among Young Women Ages 15–19

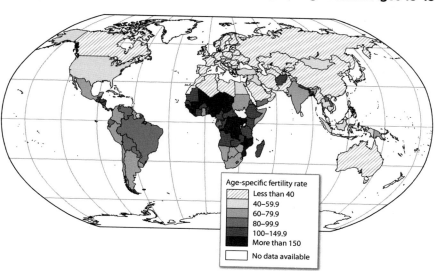

Source: United Nations Statistics Division 2013.

Conclusions

Behaviors such as smoking, alcohol and drug abuse, unhealthy eating leading to obesity, and unsafe sex leading to HIV and other sexually transmitted diseases and to underage pregnancies are prevalent in both the developed world and the developing world. These behaviors represent important threats to public health, leading to substantial mortality. Drug and alcohol use have been relatively stable over the past decade. The HIV/AIDS epidemic remains a key challenge in many developing countries, especially in Sub-Saharan Africa. However, recently the number of new infections has declined and the number of AIDS-related deaths decreased due to the scale-up of antiretroviral treatment. Smoking and obesity, traditionally associated with high-income countries, are on the rise in many developing countries. They constitute emerging threats for public health that have the potential to substantially increase mortality if they remain unaddressed.

Notes

1. At the risk of ignoring other potentially important forms of tobacco use, like bidis in India, we focus on cigarette smoking, because this is the measure most commonly collected and readily allows comparisons across countries.
2. Eriksen, Mackay, and Ross (2012) use as a source for their data the World Health Organization (WHO) report on the global tobacco epidemic (2011) and add country-specific data when missing in the WHO report.
3. A companion website to this book will include links to the full set of data used to construct the prevalence maps and tables in this chapter.
4. The Global Youth Tobacco Survey covers many countries for at least two points in time, but mainly after 2000 and only among youth, not all adults.
5. The GISAH is an Internet-based platform to display information on alcohol and health (http://www.who.int/globalatlas/alcohol). One important component of GISAH consists of the data from the Global Survey on Alcohol and Health, which was conducted from 2008. The survey data collection tool was forwarded to all WHO member states in each region for completion by focal points and national counterparts who were officially nominated by the respective ministries of health.
6. The consumption of unrecorded alcohol is associated with relatively high levels of total consumption of alcohol. Conversely, the percentage share of unrecorded alcohol consumption generally increases in regions with less total consumption (WHO 2011).
7. The WHO (2011) defines alcohol-attributable deaths as the number of deaths attributable to alcohol consumption. They assume a counterfactual scenario of no alcohol consumption. Estimates of alcohol-attributable deaths were based on population-attributable fractions for alcohol and the

number of deaths for each of the disease or injury categories. Population-attributable fractions are calculated based on the level of exposure to alcohol and the risk relations between consumption and different disease categories.

8. The indicator for patterns of drinking had been developed with optimal scaling methods based on surveys in different countries. The exact procedure is described in Rehm and others (2003).

9. See Dutta and others (2013) for an overview of the global epidemic among people who inject drugs.

References

Bonilla-Chacín, María E. 2012. *Promoting Healthy Living in Latin America and the Caribbean.* En Breve 176. Washington, DC: World Bank.

Brener, Nancy D., John O. G. Billy, and William R. Grady. 2003. "Assessment of Factors Affecting the Validity of Self-Reported Health-Risk Behavior Among Adolescents: Evidence from the Scientific Literature." *Journal of Adolescent Health* 33: 436–57.

Burkhauser, Richard V., and John Cawley. 2008. "Beyond BMI: The Value of More Accurate Measures of Fatness and Obesity in Social Science Research." *Journal of Health Economics* 27 (2): 519–29.

CDC (Centers for Diseases Control). 2013. "Teenage Pregnancy." http://www.cdc.gov/teenpregnancy.

Dutta, Arin, Andrea Wirtz, Anderson Stanciole, Robert Oelrichs, Iris Semini, Stefan Baral, Carel Pretorius, Caroline Haworth, Shannon Hader, Chris Beyrer, and Farley Cleghorn. 2013. *The Global Epidemics Among People Who Inject Drugs.* Washington, DC: World Bank. doi: 10.1596/978-0-8213-9776-3. License: Creative Commons Attribution CC BY 3.0.

Eriksen, Michael, Judith Mackay, and Hana Ross. 2012. *The Tobacco Atlas,* 4th edition. Atlanta, GA: American Cancer Society.

Hotz, V. Joseph, Charles H. Mullin, and Seth G. Sanders. 1997. "Bounding Causal Effects Using Data from a Contaminated Natural Experiment: Analysing the Effects of Teenage Childbearing." *Review of Economic Studies* 64 (4): 575–603.

Hotz, V. Joseph, Susan Williams McElroy, and Seth G. Sanders. 2005. "Teenage Childbearing and Its Life-Cycle Consequences: Exploiting a Natural Experiment." *Journal of Human Resources* 40 (3): 683–715.

INCA (Instituto Nacional de Câncer). 2010. "Global Adult Tobacco Survey: Brazil Report." INCA, Rio de Janeiro.

Institute for Health Metrics and Evaluation. 2013. "Global Burden of Disease." University of Washington, Seattle. http://www.healthmetricsandevaluation.org/gbd.

Kerrigan, Deanna, Andrea Wirtz, Stefan Baral, Michele Decker, Laura Murray, Tonia Poteat, Carel Pretorius, Susan Sherman, Mike Sweat, Iris Semini, N'Della N'Jie, Anderson Stanciole, Jenny Butler, Sutayut Osornprasop, Robert Oelrichs, and Chris Beyrer. 2013. *The Global HIV Epidemics Among Sex Workers.*

Washington, DC: World Bank. doi: 10.1596/978-0-8213-9774-9. License: Creative Commons Attribution CC BY 3.0.

Ministry of Health (Turkey). 2010. "Global Adult Tobacco Survey Turkey Report." Primary Health Care General Directorate, Ankara.

Popkin, Barry M. 2001. "The Nutrition Transition and Obesity in the Developing World." *Journal of Nutrition* 131 (3): 871S–73S.

Rehm, J., N. Rehn, R. Room, M. Monteiro, G. Gmel, D. Jernigan, and U. Frick. 2003. "The Global Distribution of Average Volume of Alcohol Consumption and Patterns of Drinking." *European Addiction Research* 9 (4): 147–56.

Shrimpton, Roger, and Claudia Rokx. 2013. "The Double Burden of Malnutrition: A Review of Global Evidence." Health, Nutrition, and Population Discussion Paper, World Bank, Washington, DC.

UNAIDS (Joint United Nations Programme on HIV/AIDS). 2012. "UNAIDS Report on the Global AIDS Epidemic." UNAIDS, Geneva.

UNFPA (United Nations Population Fund), UNAIDS (Joint United Nations Programme on HIV/AIDS), and Asia Pacific Network of Sex Workers. Forthcoming. *The HIV and Sex Work Collection: Innovative Responses in Asia and the Pacific.* Geneva: UNAIDS.

UNICEF (United Nations Children's Fund). 2008. "Young People and Family Planning: Teenage Pregnancy." UNICEF, New York.

———. 2012. *World Drug Report 2012.* New York: United Nations.

United Nations Statistics Division. 2013. "Age-Specific Fertility Rate." http://data.un.org/Data.aspx?d=GenderStat&f=inID%3A13.

United States Census Bureau. 2013. "World Population Clock Projection." http://www.census.gov/popclock.

UNODC (United Nations Office on Drugs and Crime). 2011. *World Drug Report 2011.* New York: United Nations.

WHO (World Health Organization). 2011. "Global Status Report on Alcohol and Health." WHO, Geneva, Switzerland.

———. 2013. Global Health Observatory Data Repository. http://apps.who.int/gho/data/view.main.

World Bank. 2013. World DataBank. http://databank.worldbank.org/data/home.aspx.

2

Determinants of Risky Behavior

Mattias Lundberg and Gil Shapira

Introduction

Why do individuals take risks with their health? Smoking, alcohol over-consumption, unprotected sex, and overeating are examples of behaviors that can affect the course, quality, and duration of life. These behaviors are characterized by an immediate pleasure or benefit and a long-term uncertain cost. The trade-off between the present benefit and the future costs determines the propensities of risk-taking. Whether and how individuals consider this trade-off, as well as the associated perceived benefits and costs, depend on multiple factors.

In this chapter, we explore these factors that drive people to engage in behaviors that might adversely affect their health. This includes factors that can be modified through policy interventions, as well as those that condition individual responses to policy intervention. Participation in risky health behaviors is heterogeneous: some people smoke, some people exercise, some do both. Some people are responsive to changes in prices, income, and information, while others are not. The identification of effective policies to enhance health outcomes requires that we understand what drives people to take health risks in general, what might be the impact of policies on behavior, and how we can understand the observed heterogeneity in health behaviors and policy responses.

The canonical economic model of health-related decisions derives from Grossman (1972). In the model, individuals inherit an endowment of health capital that depreciates with age but can be raised through investments. A higher stock of health capital improves productivity and earnings in addition to directly enhancing well-being. Death occurs once the health capital drops below some threshold. Forward-looking individuals make optimal health investment decisions that will maximize the expected value of lifetime welfare, which depends on health and the consumption of goods. The decisions to smoke, drink alcohol in excess, or have unprotected sex can be seen as divestments in the stock of health capital in return for a short-run increase in welfare (Cawley and Ruhm 2011). In principle, individuals consider and make trade-offs between the benefits obtained from risky and unhealthy behaviors, the costs of such behaviors, and the potentially harmful consequences for their long-term health and their life expectancy. Risk-taking depends on the weight they put on their well-being in the future relative to their well-being in the present. It is usually assumed that individuals are present-biased and discount their future well-being. The more individuals are biased toward the present, the more they are likely to take risks, regardless of the future costs and how well they understand the implications of their decisions. Furthermore, heterogeneity in health-related risk-taking arises when individuals differ in their discounting of the future.

The standard economic model exhibits some limitations in its ability to replicate empirically observed trends of behavior. These limitations do not necessarily invalidate the model, but they suggest that it is incomplete. Individuals might be constrained by the information they have, or by their ability to process and understand it. The model assumes perfect knowledge of the consequences of risky behaviors in terms of the probability and timing of potential costs. In reality, the link between current behavior and eventual outcomes is complex and depends on many factors. Individuals cannot know how the probability that they will have lung cancer in 10 years will increase if they smoke one additional cigarette. Moreover, even if individuals have perfect information, the decision-making process is complicated by the uncertainty of health outcomes, as well as the recorded habit of overestimating or underestimating likelihoods. Alternatively, the present bias is usually interpreted as discounting of the future might actually represent limited foresight. It could be that individuals do not have the capacity to project or imagine far enough into the future and accurately calculate the long-term consequences of their behavior.

Some of these behaviors, such as smoking and alcohol and drug use, are addictive. Addiction implies that the current benefit from the consumption of a substance (relative to not consuming it) depends on past consumption. With higher past consumption, greater and more frequent consumption is required to achieve the same level of satisfaction, and withdrawal from consumption decreases welfare. An influential paper by Becker and Murphy (1988) lays out a rational model of addiction and portrays the implications regarding the effect of prices on consumption. In their model, forward-looking individuals might make an optimal choice to consume an addictive substance, although they know that their current consumption will cause addiction.

Orphanides and Zervos (1995) propose a modified model of addiction, in which individuals are uncertain about the addictive power of the substances they consume. With consumption, individuals update their subjective beliefs about the costs of their behavior. Conditional on their subjective beliefs, though, individuals are forward-looking and making decisions that would maximize their perceived lifetime welfare. Individuals in the model might regret their past behavior, which is shown to be prevalent among addicts. Slovic (2001), for example, has found that more than 85 percent of adult smokers say they would not start smoking if they could "do it all over again," and that this feeling was even stronger among those who had tried many times to quit. Although the Orphanides and Zervos model is less strict than that of Becker and Murphy, the capacity of addicts to make rational decisions can be questioned, especially when making decisions under the influence of alcohol or drugs. In any case, it is reasonable to expect addiction to limit individuals' responses to different policy interventions, at least in the short term.

This chapter also presents evidence that behavior is conditioned by fundamental individual characteristics that are partly biological, psychological, and social. As we show, preferences and manifest behavior are highly sensitive to context, mood, and short-term physiological changes, especially hormonal. Preferences and behavior are contingent and inseparable, depending on previous behavior, regret, and disappointment, as much as individuals may be forward-looking; even if they are forward-looking, people can exhibit wildly inconsistent preferences over time, and fail to accurately estimate both the ability to change behaviors and the consequences of their actions.

We explore different factors that are theorized or shown to affect propensities to engage in health-related risky behavior. Where possible, we place greater emphasis on evidence from low- and middle-income countries; however, some of the factors are global rather than specific to wealth or culture. We also acknowledge that the division of the chapter into different sections is based on convenience rather than theory. Some of these factors interact, and some are partly endogenous to others. It is also important to stress that we do not attempt to provide an exhaustive review of all the relevant literature.

Empirically identifying the impact of each of the different potential determinants of risky behaviors is challenging.

- First, different determinants might be correlated. For example, if we are interested in measuring the effect of wealth on propensity to engage in a certain behavior, a wealthy person is more likely to have a higher level of schooling and belong to different social networks than a poorer person. If education and social norms also affect behavior, it is difficult to separate the influence of these multiple potential factors that drive behavior.
- Second, unobservable factors might affect both risk-taking as well as some of the potential determinants of risky behaviors. The relationship between education and risk-taking is one example. Investments in education and avoidance of risk-taking both involve a trade-off between current costs or benefits and future well-being, and they can both be affected by factors such as self-control and impatience. Wealth itself requires investments and savings, which require some appreciation of the value of the future as well.
- Conversely, an observed association between different factors and risk-taking may be coincidental rather than causal.

In the discussion that follows, we prioritize research that is taking into account these empirical challenges. However, even when causality cannot be proven, understanding associations between different factors and risk-taking can be helpful in better targeting policy interventions to different groups.

Education

There are several direct and indirect pathways through which education is theorized to both increase and decrease engagement in health-related risky behaviors. Better-educated individuals might not only have better access to health-related information but also have better ability to process that information (Grossman 1972). Understanding the causality between current actions and future health outcomes might result in safer behavior. A higher level of education can also translate into better job opportunities. Perceptions of higher income, consumption, and well-being in the future might increase present valuation of being alive in the future and promote caution (Becker 1993). Another potential pathway is through social networks, if behaviors of others influence one's own behavior. The composition of the social network is partly determined by one's peers in school and at work. In addition, better-educated individuals, especially in developing countries, enjoy greater geographical mobility, which can make them less influenced by local social norms. Education may also affect engagement in risky behaviors through determining income, in ways that will be discussed.

Education and Smoking

Studies show that a college education has a negative impact on smoking in the United States. This literature serves as a good example of how researchers approached the challenge of identifying the causal effect of education on a risky behavior using different econometric methods. These studies start with an observation that lower levels of education are strongly correlated with smoking. Farrell and Fuchs (1982) use data about the retrospective smoking histories of Californian men and women who completed high school. They are able to link smoking behavior at age 17, when the entire sample was in high school, to smoking and education attainment at age 24. They find that those who smoked when in high school attained lower levels of education relative to those who did not. The reported smoking behaviors during high school years lead the authors to reject the hypothesis that college education causes differences in smoking in favor of a hypothesis that unobservable factors influence smoking and schooling simultaneously. Using similar types of data, but from a nationally representative sample and exploiting a longer time frame, de Walque (2010) concludes that college education has a negative effect on smoking in women. He also shows that, although there is an overall decrease in smoking prevalence, better-educated individuals were quicker to respond to information about the dangers of smoking after such information became available, beginning in the 1950s.

Other studies applied the instrumental variables approach to recover the effect of education on smoking; these studies exploit factors they claim have affected the level of individuals' education but could have only affected smoking through the change in education level. Therefore, the response in smoking to the change in education can be attributed to education and not to a latent factor that might affect both education and smoking simultaneously. Sander (1995a, 1995b) employs family background characteristics, Currie and Moretti (2003) exploit variations in the availability of colleges in women's counties when they were age 17, and de Walque (2007a) makes use of the draft during the Vietnam War that caused individuals to enroll in college to avoid military service. All of these studies find negative effects of education on smoking.[1]

A related study from a different setting is Jensen and Lleras-Muney (2012). The authors use data from a randomized intervention, which provided information to male teenagers on the returns to schooling, without additional health benefits information. Those exposed to the intervention completed more years of schooling and were less likely to work in the four years following the intervention. In addition, the teens in the treatment group were less likely to smoke and consume alcohol. The authors attribute the effect of schooling on these risky behaviors to exposure to different peer groups. In addition, those who attend school and do not work have less disposable income to spend on cigarettes and alcohol.[2]

Education and HIV Risk

Studies of the relationship between education and HIV risk in Sub-Saharan Africa have reached different conclusions, suggesting this relationship might depend on other factors and evolve over time.[3] Curiously, the discordance between these studies is not about whether education is a cause of risk-taking or risk-avoidance, but whether there is an association between education and HIV infection. Studies investigating this relationship consider both reported sexual behavior as well as actual HIV infection, a consequence of risky behavior, as indicators of interest. It is important to keep in mind that HIV infection is only a proxy for engagement in risky sexual behavior because risky sex does not necessarily result in infection. First, individuals might have practiced unsafe sex with HIV-negative individuals. Second, even if the partner is infected, the average transmission probability from a single sexual encounter with an infected person is estimated to be less than 1 percent.[4] In addition, some might choose a low level of risk, by having a single partner, for example, but be exposed to the risk of infection through unobserved behaviors of their sexual partners. Finally, self-reported sexual behavior is often biased.

Several studies have concluded that there is a positive association between schooling levels and HIV infection. Smith and others (1999), for example, find such relationship using data from the Rakai district of rural Uganda. However, when the analysis is stratified by place of residence, the association holds only for rural villages and not for trading centers. Later studies have exploited nationally representative Demographic and Health Surveys (DHS) data that included HIV testing of respondents. Using such data from five countries, Fortson (2008) finds that more educated individuals are more likely to be infected with HIV and that education is correlated with premarital sex.

In contrast, de Walque (2009) uses the same data as Fortson (2008) and controls jointly for education and wealth. He concludes that education is not positively or negatively associated with HIV status. However, he does find that schooling is an important determinant of related behaviors and knowledge. On the one hand, individuals with higher levels of schooling are more likely to report condom use and are more knowledgeable about the epidemic. On the other hand, these protective practices might be offset by the fact that individuals with higher levels of education are more likely to engage in extramarital sex and are less likely to practice abstinence.

Some papers have suggested that the mixed results are due to actual heterogeneity in the association between education and HIV across populations and over time (for example, de Walque and Kline 2011; Fortson 2008). De Walque (2007b) shows a change in the HIV/education gradient for young females in rural Uganda. In 1990, when relatively little was known about the epidemic, there was no association between HIV infection and education. In 2000, however, more educated women were less likely to be infected. The study also shows that condom use is more prevalent among women with higher schooling levels and concludes that education increases responsiveness to information campaigns.

Iorio and Santaeulalia-Llopis (2011) exploit DHS data from 18 Sub-Saharan countries and describe a U-shape pattern of the HIV/education gradient over time. Education is positively correlated with HIV prevalence in early stages of the epidemic in the different countries, but this relationship disappears with time. The reason for the initial positive correlation, according to the authors, is that individuals with more schooling have more sexual partners. Nevertheless, better-educated persons are more likely to acquire information about how to avoid HIV infection and to change their behavior. Interestingly, the authors also find that as the epidemic matures, the positive association between HIV and education reappears. The authors attribute that trend to better access to antiretroviral treatment by educated individuals. Although they are less likely to be newly infected, the rate of infection among them increases because they survive longer once infected.

Wealth and Income

Wealth, like education, can affect risk-taking through multiple, potentially opposing, mechanisms. This section considers jointly the roles of wealth (stock) and income (flow) in affecting risk-taking. As with education, there are numerous potential mechanisms through which wealth and income might either increase or decrease risk-taking. Above all, individuals with more resources can afford to consume more commodities and services, including risky ones such as alcohol, cigarettes, and transactional sex. From the perspective of consumer choice theory, additional income can either increase or decrease consumption of risky goods, depending on the consumers' relative valuation of all goods. For example, additional income might cause a household to shift from purchasing unhealthy food to purchasing healthier but more expensive food. Another way through which wealth might affect risk-taking is through better access to health services, which, in turn, affects exposure to health information. Access to health services could also mitigate the harmful consequences of risky behavior, altering the trade-off between current benefit and future cost. For example, access to antiretroviral treatment can potentially reduce the perceived cost of being HIV-infected and therefore increase unsafe sexual behavior. Some of the pathways through which wealth can affect risky behavior are similar to those described in the preceding section on education. Wealth might promote safer behavior because wealthier individuals might be less willing to risk their perceived high level of well-being in the future. Wealth status might also affect the composition of social networks and increase geographical mobility. Lastly, individuals from wealthier backgrounds are more likely to be sent to school as children, which can affect behaviors.

Income Elasticity of Demand for Risky Goods

Evidence suggests that higher income is associated with greater consumption of risky goods such as cigarettes and alcohol. Many have studied the relationships between income and consumption of alcohol, cigarettes, and unhealthy food. In particular, a large economic literature focuses on the measurement of the income elasticity of demand for cigarettes and alcohol, that is, by how much the amount demanded of a good changes when income increases but prices remain fixed. Meta-analyses of this literature document that these elasticities are, on average, positive (Gallet 2007; Gallet and List 2003). Although the studies find, on average, that an increase in income is associated with a rise in demand for these risky goods, they also record a large variation in the estimated elasticities, driven by the different methods and different types of data used for the calculation.

Wealth, Income Shocks, and HIV Risk

Although no clear relationship exists between wealth status and HIV risk in Sub-Saharan Africa, income shocks have been shown to affect exposure to risk of infection through transactional sex. The association between wealth and HIV has been the focus of several studies, which, like the related studies on the education/HIV gradient, resulted in diverging conclusions. Mishra and others (2007) analyze DHS data from eight Sub-Saharan African countries and conclude that individuals in the wealthiest quintiles are more likely to be HIV-infected in each of the countries included in their study. Other studies, however, maintain that there is not a consistent pattern across or even within countries and that the wealth/HIV gradient changes when different measures of wealth are used (Beegle and de Walque 2009; Fortson 2008). Gillespie, Kadiyala, and Greener (2007), in a review of studies exploring this relationship, suggest that the relationship between HIV and wealth might be dynamic and evolving.

In the context of the HIV/AIDS epidemic in Sub-Saharan Africa, several studies have described how poverty and income shocks influence sexual behaviors in general and engagement in transactional sex in particular. These studies often describe a market in which men demand sex, for which they are willing to pay with money or gifts, and women supply it. Following this simplistic description of the environment, the number of sexual partners a man has is expected to increase with wealth or as a result of a positive income shock. For women, the prediction is that engagement in transactional sex will increase with a negative economic shock. The overall impact of aggregate income shocks, which affect communities and not just individual households, is ambiguous, since they have opposing effects on the willingness of men and women to engage in such practices.

Dinkelman, Lam, and Leibbrandt (2007, 2008) find that wealth is associated with later sexual debut for young females in Cape Town, South Africa. They also find that both young men and women are more likely to have multiple partnerships after experiencing a negative economic shock. The shocks considered in these studies are negative economic shocks at the household level, such as a death of a household member, job loss, or a loss of support from outside of the household. Kohler and Thornton (2012) assess the impact of a conditional cash transfer program in Malawi, in which individuals received a transfer if they maintain their HIV status for a year. Although the program was not found to affect HIV status or reported sexual behavior by participants, the transfers received at the end of the implementation of the policy experiment affected subsequent behaviors. Men who received the transfers were more likely, and women were less likely, to report engaging in risky sexual behavior.

Robinson and Yeh (2011, 2012) analyze a unique dataset constructed from self-reported diaries of 192 sex workers in western Kenya. They find that the women increase the quantity of transactional sex they supply in response to health shocks incurred in the household (Robinson and Yeh 2011). Moreover, they supply riskier sex, which is better compensated, in response to these shocks. The diaries also show that women develop long-term relationships with regular clients who provide transfers after the women suffer negative income shocks (Robinson and Yeh 2012). In sum, these studies show that engagement in risky sex is a means for women in western Kenya to smooth consumption in response to shocks, and that development of longer-term relationships with clients serves as an insurance mechanism against potential future shocks.

Several studies explored the effect of aggregate income shocks on the spread of HIV. Burke, Gong, and Jones (2012) link biomarker data on the HIV status of individuals to measures of rainfall in 19 Sub-Saharan African countries. In this context, variation in rainfall represents an important driver of variation in income. Exposure to such aggregate income shocks is shown to lead to a significant increase in overall infection, concentrated in rural areas, which are more affected. Several potential behavioral reactions to the income shocks might bring an increase in HIV incidence. The authors show that their results are consistent with an increase in transactional sex and are less consistent with changes in sexual behaviors due to migration or early sexual debut of young women who drop out of school. Exposure to shocks significantly increases the probability that individuals will have multiple partners. Moreover, the effect is larger for women working in the agricultural sector, who are more likely to be affected by the change in rainfall. For men, the effect is bigger for those who do not work in agriculture and are therefore less likely to be affected.

Relatedly, Wilson (2012) examines the effect of a positive aggregate economic shock, a sudden surge in copper production in Zambia in the early 2000s. The analysis exploits the increase in copper production, as well as its variation across mining cities, and finds that the increased production brought reductions in transactional sex and multiple partnerships. The author concludes that the opportunities for women to gain income outside that derived from transactional sex dominated the increased demand for sex by men.

Prices

Prices decrease consumption because they represent an immediate and certain cost, unlike the future and uncertain health consequences that individuals might incur from engaging in health-related risky behaviors. In the standard economic model, an increase in the price of a normal good results in a fall in consumption. Therefore, even if myopia and intense discounting of the future drive the engagements in risky behaviors, individuals are expected to alter their consumption when prices change. The effect of a price change on the consumption of risky goods is especially of interest, since price manipulation, mostly through taxing, is a common policy lever used by governments as discussed in more detail in chapter 5.

The responsiveness of consumption to price changes might be limited if the decision making regarding the consumption of goods such as cigarettes and alcohol is influenced by habit formation or addiction. The estimation of the price elasticity of demand for these substances has been the focus of many studies; the researchers estimated the change in consumption given a change in the price of the substance, all else being fixed. In addition to the many studies on the topic are numerous meta-analyses and review papers summarizing this literature.[5] These studies employ different types of data (individual or aggregate level) and use different econometric models.

Overall, although there is a variation in the estimated elasticities, this literature provides strong evidence that consumption of cigarettes and alcohol falls when their prices increase. With respect to smoking, it is also shown that the long-run price elasticity of demand is greater than the short-run elasticity. This trend implies that the response to the change in price might be gradual, at least for some consumers.

Price of Unsafe Sex

Studies in different settings have shown that unsafe sex with sex workers is associated with a higher price paid by the clients. The clients' willingness to pay more implies a higher satisfaction from unprotected sex. From the point of view of the sex workers, this example is different than the ones discussed because exposure to risk depends on the price received by the woman, and not paid by her. However, as in the other examples, the price changes the trade-off between the current benefit and the future cost. A challenge in estimating the compensation differential for condom use is that the association between unprotected sex and price might not represent causality. It could be that the difference in price is due to sorting of clients or unobservable characteristics of the sex workers that affect their preferences for condom use and their ability to bargain for price simultaneously. Rao and others (2003) evaluate the compensation differential for condom use among sex workers in Calcutta, India. The authors exploit a nonsystematic provision of safe sex information to sex workers, which increased the propensity of the women to use condoms but should have not affected their ability to bargain or the clients' willingness to pay for their services. The study finds that sex workers who use condoms are facing an estimated loss of income of between 66 and 79 percent. Gertler, Shah, and Bertozzi (2005) employ a different econometric strategy by analyzing a panel dataset that contains information on several of the most recent transactions by sex workers in two Mexican states. Having the information on several transactions for each sex worker allows the authors to control for the women's fixed unobservable characteristics, which might impact condom use and price jointly. They estimate a 23 percent premium for not using a condom. Robinson and Yeh (2011), with the data described previously, employ a similar estimation strategy and find a lower premium of 7.8 percent in Busia, Kenya.

Life Expectancy and Competing Risks

If individuals assign a low likelihood to being healthy or alive in the future, the cost of engaging in a risky behavior might seem limited or even negligible. Individuals in low-income countries suffer from high rates of morbidity and mortality from multiple sources, as well as low access to quality health services. A number of papers explore the relationship between longevity and investments in human capital, both theoretically and empirically.[6] Dow, Philipson, and Sala-i-Martin (1999) develop a theoretical model of investments in health in an environment of competing health risks. They show empirically that a health policy targeting one health risk can bring an increase in investments by individuals to prevent other causes of death. Specifically, they find that the Expanded Programme on Immunization of the United Nations significantly increased birth weight, even though there is no direct biological effect of the immunization on birth weight.

Viewing engagement in risky behaviors as divestment in health, the existence of competing health risks might also affect propensities of risk-taking. Oster (2012) explores whether life expectancy without HIV infection affects responsiveness to the HIV risk, using regional child and maternal mortality as well as malaria prevalence rates as proxies for non-HIV life expectancy. She finds that individuals living in areas with high non-HIV mortality are less likely to reduce risky sexual behavior in response to local HIV prevalence. This finding accords with the theoretical framework suggested by Dow and others (1999).

Information and Beliefs

Individuals make decisions given their perceptions of the environment, which might not accurately represent the actual environment. For example, individuals might not be aware of the future consequences of risky behaviors. The studies about smoking in the United States and sexual behavior in the context of the HIV/AIDS epidemic in Sub-Saharan Africa suggest that behavior did change after information became available about risks of smoking and the transmission of HIV. Kenkel (1991) shows that health knowledge explains part of the difference in the consumption of cigarettes, alcohol, and exercising observed in individuals with different levels of schooling in the United States. The study also shows, however, that individuals who are knowledgeable about the negative consequences of these behaviors will also engage in them.

Even if individuals are aware of the potential negative consequences, they might have misperceptions about the likelihood of or the severity with which these consequences will affect them. Awareness and subjective expectations can alter the perceived trade-off between the benefit and costs associated with risky behaviors in ways that can increase or decrease engagement. For example, many young people who begin to smoke see few health risks from smoking the next cigarette or even from smoking regularly for a few years. They tend also to overestimate their own ability to stop smoking; above all, smokers do not understand how their future selves will regret the original decision to begin smoking (Slovic 2000, 2001).

Research around the AIDS epidemic suggests that people will change their behavior in response to perceived risks of infection and illness. Expectations of the evolution of the epidemic and future medical treatments can affect current behavior (de Walque, Kazianga, and Over. 2012). This dynamic can have counterintuitive consequences. For example, people may not engage in much protective behavior during the initial stages of an epidemic, not only because current risk is minimal, but also because they correctly anticipate that the epidemic will get worse over time; pessimistic expectations can thus increase the pace of epidemic transmission (Auld 2003). Crepaz, Hart, and Marks (2004) found that beliefs about the availability and effectiveness of treatment can actually increase the temptation to have unprotected sex. Similarly, the introduction of two fake but perceived effective cures for AIDS, Kemron and Pearl Omega, led to a drop in condom use among sex workers in Kenya (Jha and others 2001).

An HIV-infected person can live for years without experiencing any symptoms, even without any treatment (Morgan and others 2002). Without testing, one's own status is uncertain, as long as there is or has been exposure to risk. There is a possibly circular relationship between beliefs and behaviors in infectious diseases: behaviors can affect beliefs about infection, and beliefs can affect behaviors. Moreover, the way in which beliefs about infection affect behaviors is ambiguous. On the one hand, individuals who believe they are highly likely to be infected might reduce their incentive to protect themselves. On the other hand, individuals may want to avoid infecting others. Using longitudinal data from rural Malawi, Delavande and Kohler (2012) find that the decisions to engage in risky sex and the likelihood of having multiple partners depend on individuals' perceived probabilities of their own and their partners' HIV status, their expectations about the HIV transmission rate, and their expectations about how HIV infection affects survival. Using the same dataset, De Paula and others (forthcoming) find that an increase in the perceived likelihood of infection is associated with a decrease in the likelihood of engaging in extramarital sex. Gong (2011) exploits a randomized trial conducted in Kenya and Tanzania in which a treatment group received voluntary counseling and testing while the control group only received health information. He finds that individuals who believed that they were unlikely to be infected but received a positive test result were more likely to contract sexually transmitted diseases after the test. In this case, an increase in the perceived likelihood of being infected increased the propensity to engage in risky sex.

Risk Compensation

Some evidence supports the idea that when individuals are able to reduce risks in one area, they might choose to increase risk-taking in another (Peltzman 1975). This means that investments to decrease some specific risks associated with a certain behavior may actually have limited or no effect on the overall risks associated with that behavior. Drivers in the United States responded to the introduction of mandatory seatbelt laws and the installation of antilock braking systems and airbags in cars by driving more quickly, thereby reducing some of the benefits obtained by the safety innovations (Wilde 2002). It must be noted that these safety innovations have significantly decreased deaths among the occupants in cars involved in traffic accidents, even though they may have not reduced the incidence of traffic accidents. These compensating risks can overwhelm the intended benefits of technologies or policies intended to enhance health or safety, especially if the effects on others are considered. Evidence indicates that seatbelt laws have led to increased fatalities among motorcyclists, pedestrians, and bicyclists struck by cars (Vrolix 2006). Risk compensation may differ between men and women; one study found that speeds increased among male cyclists but not among female cyclists after the introduction of rules mandating helmet use (Messiah and others 2012).

Psychological Determinants of Risk-Taking

Individual choices, behaviors, and responses to prices, incomes, and other signals are determined by fundamental individual characteristics, beliefs, and perceptions of the world. Individual differences in behavior and risk-taking are usually regarded as arising from differences in fundamental characteristics that describe what those individuals believe about themselves and the world, such as probabilities and preferences over risks and time, and behavioral traits that describe how they act, such as self-control. Loewenstein and O'Donoghue (2004) refer to the *deliberative* and *affective* systems of decision making; the first involves foresight, intention, and planning, and the second is reactive and impulsive.[7] In the deliberative system, individuals are more likely to account properly for future costs and to control urges; in the affective system, they are more likely to yield to desires, possibly even against their better judgments. The following section describes the different characteristics that influence choices and responses.

Discounting

Many of the behaviors described here bring short-term pleasures at the expense of costs that are both in the future and stochastic. Most people discount the future, whether future gains or losses. Many people exhibit hyperbolic discounting, in which preferences are always biased toward the more immediate rewards, regardless of how they understand the consequences in the long term, even if they understand that their future selves would prefer the safer outcome. Alternatively, they may have limited foresight. Regardless of bias or impatience, people cannot project or imagine far enough into the future to understand what the long-term consequences of their behavior really are.

In general, discount rates are a significant predictor of health-related behavior and saving decisions. Using standard choice list tasks, Sutter and others (2010) find that more impatient children and adolescents are more likely to spend money on alcohol and cigarettes, have a higher body mass index (BMI), and are less likely to save money. Higher discount rates are also significantly associated among youth with heavier alcohol consumption and the frequency of drunkenness (Bishai 2001; Vuchinich and Simpson 1998); as well as a range of sexual behaviors, including ever having sex, having sex before age 16 years, and past or current pregnancy (Chesson and others 2006). Bishai (2004) shows that impatience also falls with age.

Impulsivity

Discounting and impatience are related to self-control and impulsivity. Some people are more impulsive than others, but the ability to control impulsive behavior and resist temptation varies across domains within individuals much more than it varies among individuals. Impulsive people can exhibit both patience and impatience, and more importantly, people can be overwhelmed by desires even though they understand and properly value the future consequences. Impulsivity is relatively stable across time, although children exhibit more impulsivity than older people. A 40-year study by Casey and others (2011) shows that preschoolers who were able to delay gratification were more likely to be able to do so in their twenties, thirties, and forties. Individuals develop cognitive and behavioral tools early on to help them deal with temptation. In a series of celebrated experiments (Mischel and Mendoza-Denton 2003), it was shown that preschool children have sophisticated strategies to avoid eating marshmallows, and that those who can control their immediate desires for marshmallows go on to receive more education and obtain higher test scores than others. Conversely, other studies have shown that those who are unable to delay gratification are much more likely to consume tobacco, marijuana, and alcohol (Romer and others 2010), and to be obese. (Seeyave and others 2009). Impulsive behavior is motivated by rewards more than by harm; in other words, those who behave impulsively are much more influenced by the perceived benefits of the behavior than they are dissuaded by their assessment of the harm associated with it (Tsukayama and others n.d.). There is an interesting link between impulsivity and the *perception* of time: in one experiment, impulsive subjects overestimated the duration of time intervals, and accordingly they discounted the value of delayed rewards even more strongly than self-controlled individuals (Wittmann and Paulus 2007).

Most people have a limited and easily exhausted capacity for self-control. Evidence suggests that exerting self-control in one domain can make it more difficult to exercise self-control in other domains. For instance, suppressing emotions diminishes physical stamina, and stress decreases cognitive control (Baumeister and others 1994; Liston, McEwen, and Casey 2009; Muraven, Tice, and Baumeister 1998). In one frequently cited study, Shiv and Fedorikhin (1999) found that people asked to perform a mentally taxing task were more likely to choose chocolate cake than fruit salad. Spears (2010) conducted similar experiments with groups in India and the United States and concluded that poverty interferes with the ability to exercise control and make effective decisions. Among poor people, managing day-to-day existence is sufficiently demanding in terms of cognitive resources that it impedes deliberative and goal-seeking behavior. Banerjee and Mullainathan (2010) argue that this observation may, in part, explain the "wasted expenditure" observed among poor people, whether in terms of savings and investments or in terms of drinking and smoking.

Early Life Experiences

Evidence indicates that early life experiences can influence risk-taking throughout life. Children's willingness to take risks is strongly associated with their parents' willingness to take risks in many domains, including driving, career choices, and health behavior (Falk 2012). Adverse early-life circumstances, stress, and subsequent post-traumatic stress disorder can lead to increased risk-taking (Bremner 2005). The adverse childhood events (ACE) study interviewed over 17,000 adults to examine the link between childhood experience and adult health. The number of self-reported adverse childhood events is positively correlated with risks for smoking, alcohol abuse, illicit drug use, sexually transmitted diseases, suicide attempts, early sexual debut, and early pregnancy (Felitti and Anda 2005; Middlebrooks and Audage 2008).

Studies of children who have been exposed to war or other violent conflict have repeatedly shown significantly higher incidences of anxiety, depression, and lower self-confidence, especially among those who had perpetrated violence (Betancourt 2010). Joseph and others (2006) find that children who are exposed to violence in early life are more likely to have friends who smoke, drink alcohol, and use illicit drugs; this likelihood does not extend to the children themselves. Conversely, drug use and easy access to them can lead to violence. Adolescents who report greater drug or alcohol use, either their own or in the immediate community, are more likely to have been victims of violence. It may be that drug use impairs judgment and the ability to recognize cues of impending violence (Morojele and Brook 2006). The Minnesota Longitudinal Study of Risk and Adaptation found that a harsh and unpredictable early life (ages 0 to 5) was a strong predictor of both sexual and other risk-taking behavior at age 23. Individuals exposed to more unpredictable, rapidly changing environments during the first five years of life had more sexual partners, engaged in more aggressive and delinquent behaviors, and were more likely to be associated with criminal activities (Simpson and others 2012). Cardoso and Verner (2008) found that living in a violent home has a significant detrimental impact on the use of drugs, increasing their consumption.

Data from developing and developed countries show that orphans are more likely to make riskier choices than non-orphans (Thurman and others 2006). One study in Northern Mali showed that orphanhood is a significant predictor of age at first sex. Males whose parents both died report having experienced first sexual intercourse earlier than their male non-orphan peers. Similarly, female maternal and paternal orphans had their sexual debut faster than their non-orphan counterparts (Mkandawire, Tenkorang, and Luginaah 2012). A review of studies on HIV risk in orphaned populations, which primarily includes samples from Sub-Saharan Africa, shows orphaned youth are twice as likely to be HIV positive and to have higher levels of sexual risk behavior than their non-orphaned peers (Operario and others 2011). However, a study from Nyanza, Kenya, did not find a link between orphanhood and risky sexual behavior (Juma and others 2013).

Social Determinants of Risk-Taking

Choices are also social; our behaviors and even our preferences reflect the behaviors of those around us, and our settings determine the risks to which we are potentially exposed (Fehr 2009). Norms are the rules that govern behaviors within the group; they may be prescriptive and codified into established laws, or they may be more informal (Cialdini and Trost 1998). They establish what one "should" do and encourage compliance through reinforcement or sanction.

Norms and Networks

From the early days of the HIV/AIDS pandemic, there has been a clear understanding of the importance of networks in spreading the disease.

The disease appeared to spread, among other places, along trunk roads and major shipment networks. Research into the sexual networks of truck drivers in Nigeria (Orubuloye, Caldwell, and Caldwell 1993), South Africa (Varga 2001), Uganda (Pickering and others 1997), Bangladesh (Gibney, Saquib, and Metzger 2003), China (Yang and others 2010), and many other places revealed that the disease followed trucking patterns. Part of the reason for the spread had to do with the number of concurrent partnerships among truck drivers and their partners along the route, as well as the inconsistent and generally low incidence of condom use. Truck drivers surveyed in Nigeria had on average six regular partners, one at each of their overnight stops. About half of the young market women surveyed at those stops report regularly supplementing their income by providing sex for money (Orubuloye and others 1993). In Bangladesh, truck drivers reported having five partners during the previous year; moreover, of the 343 subjects in the Bangladesh study who reported having sexual intercourse, fewer than one-third had *ever* used a condom, and most of those subjects had used a condom only once or occasionally (Gibney, Saquib, and Metzger 2003).

High rates of HIV infection were also found among others who engaged in similarly circulatory migration for work. HIV prevalence has been higher among some fishing communities in low- and middle-income countries. Most of the studies supporting this claim speculate that the mobile and migratory nature of fish-catching operations increases susceptibility to HIV exposure (Kissling and others 2005). Miners in southern Africa were among the drivers of the early AIDS epidemic, moving from the mines, where male miners lived apart from their spouses and were exposed to high-risk sex, back to their families, to whom they brought the infection (see, for example, Lurie and others 1997).

Norms may change over time and experience, and they may differ by individual characteristics, such as education or wealth. Huebner and others (2011) found that attitudes toward unprotected anal intercourse changed as a function of previous behavior, as if we adjust our standards to suit our behavior rather than the other way around. Norms and manifest behavior change with the reference group and network, and there is strong evidence that networks influence obesity (Christakis and Fowler 2007), smoking (Christakis and Fowler 2008), intravenous drug use (Latkin and others 2010), and contraceptive behavior (Kincaid 2000). A study among adolescents in Cape Town, South Africa, finds that peer pressure among both boys and girls undermines healthy social norms and the impact of HIV prevention messages to abstain, be faithful, use condoms, and delay sexual debut (Selikow and others 2009). However, a study among sex workers in the Dominican Republic finds that condom use is higher among male clients with tighter social networks (Barrington and others 2009). The celebrated Framingham Heart Study found that the decision to quit smoking was highly correlated within well-defined clusters: the average size of smoking clusters remained constant as the prevalence of smoking declined, implying that entire clusters stopped at the same time. Smoking cessation by a spouse decreased a person's chances of smoking by 67 percent, and smoking cessation by a friend decreased the chances by 36 percent (Christakis and Fowler 2008).

Context also influences self-control. Especially among adolescents, the presence of peers increases risk-taking by heightening sensitivity to the potential reward value of risky decisions. Being around friends increases sensation-seeking behavior (Barbalat and others 2010). Gardner and Steinberg (2005) randomly assigned young people to engage in a simulated driving task alone or in the presence of two friends. They found that participants took more risks, focused more on the benefits than the costs of risky behavior, and made riskier decisions when in peer groups than alone; the peer effects on risk-taking and risky decision making were stronger among adolescents and youths than adults. Adolescents took a substantially greater number of risks when observed by peers. This is borne out strongly in the observational data. In the United States, accident rates among novice teenage drivers were 75 percent lower in the presence of adult passengers and 96 percent higher among those teenagers driving with risky friends (Simons-Morton and others 2011).

Although the influence of context and network suggests that risk-taking behavior can be manipulated by changing the environment, the evidence of this is limited. One study of the "Moving to Opportunity" program in the United States, which enabled poor families to move out of poor neighborhoods, found that females in families that received vouchers and counseling experienced improvements in education and mental health and were less likely to engage in risky behaviors; females in families that received only vouchers experienced improvements in mental health. Males in both treatment groups were more likely than controls to engage in risky behaviors and to experience physical health problems (Kling and Liebman 2004).[8]

Social Capital

The majority of evidence suggests a positive correlation between social engagement and healthy behavior. Pronyk and others (2008) observed in South Africa that greater social capital was associated with safer reported behavior and lower risk-taking in general; it was also associated with higher rates of HIV infection. A long-term study in northwestern Tanzania showed that social engagement may be related to fewer sexual partners, a higher probability of monogamous relationships, less casual sex, and greater condom use (Frumence and others 2011). Cardoso and Verner (2008) find that teenagers in Brazil who stated that they rely on friends' support are less likely to use drugs, while reliance on people in the neighborhood seems to be associated with a lower probability of teen pregnancy.

Growing up in violent and unstable communities can lead to an increase in risk-taking behavior. Cardoso and Verner (2008) also find that young people in violent communities in Brazil are more likely to engage in other risky behaviors. Similarly, in a fascinating set of field experiments in rural Burundi, Voors and others (2012) also find that individuals exposed to violence are more risk-seeking and have higher discount rates.

Biological Determinants of Risk-Taking

Attitudes and preferences toward risk and risk-taking are partly encoded in our genes and in our fundamental physiological development, and they are influenced heavily by biological processes and changes over the life-cycle. The impact of policies designed to influence risk-taking will vary across individuals depending on specific genetically encoded characteristics, as well as on their age and experience. Understanding these differences may lead to more sharply targeted and specifically effective interventions, for example, among adolescents.

Studies that have tried to separate the influence of various attributes suggest that as much as half of the variation in risk preferences can be explained by genetic factors (Zyphur and others 2009). Stoel and others (2006) found that "sensation-seeking" is inherited from one generation to the next, and is much stronger in pairs of identical (monozygotic) twins than in fraternal (dizygotic) twins. Greater risk-taking and shorter time preference are correlated strongly with genetic markers that limit the uptake of certain neurotransmitters such as dopamine in the brain (Carpenter, Garcia, and Koji Lum 2011).[9] Those that possess this trait require greater stimulation to feel the same sensation from dopamine (Dreber and others 2010); and this is also associated with differences in sexual desire, arousal, and behavior (Ben Zion and others 2006). In addition, the expression of genetically coded traits can itself be influenced by experience in a process known as *epigenesis*. For example, antenatal exposure to testosterone, which is produced by stress, is a significant predictor of risk and time preferences, particularly among males (Drichoutis and Nayga 2012).

Physiological Development

Much of what is considered dangerously risky behavior begins in adolescence. Despite generally outstanding physical health, the risk of injury or death during adolescence is 2–3 times that of childhood. The primary cause of this increase in morbidity and mortality is heightened risky behavior. Moreover, the habits that are formed during this period largely determine health outcomes later in life. Smoking, unprotected sex, and excessive alcohol consumption are not immediately deadly; the consequences are manifest much later than the behavior. Cigarette smoking peaked in the United States in 1945; deaths from lung cancer did not peak until 30 years later, in the 1970s and 1980s (Centers for Disease Control and Prevention 1993).

Adolescence is a time of experimentation and identity formation, and this process is as much biological as social. The brain evolves in stages throughout childhood and adolescence. The greater prevalence of risk-taking behavior among adolescents partly arises from delays in executive function, including judgment, impulse control, self-monitoring, and planning, all of which develop more slowly than the desire for stimulation and sensation (Pharo and others 2011; Steinberg 2008). In adolescence, the incentive-processing, reward-seeking part of the brain grows rapidly (Steinberg 2008). The parts of the brain involved in active cognitive judgment and control—that govern the capacity for self-regulation and self-control—develop more gradually, through at least the mid-twenties (Giedd 2008).

Another consequence of uneven brain development is that although people are generally more sensitive to loss than gain, adolescents are less averse to losses than adults and are more sensitive to reward. They are much more attracted by the "high" or euphoria than they are worried about the prospect of punishment or loss, and much more so than adults (Barbalat and others 2010). All adolescents, but especially those who are predisposed to impatience, will fail to project future costs and benefits (Fareri, Martin, and Delgado 2008). Thus, information campaigns that highlight the potential costs of risky behavior will be less effective among adolescents, even if they understand the consequences in principle.

Early maturation, and especially the early onset of menarche in girls, is correlated with greater risk-taking in sexual and other behavior. Downing and Bellis (2009) found that girls experiencing earlier puberty are more likely to drink alcohol, be drunk, smoke, and use drugs before the age of 14; they are also more likely to have a sexual debut and unprotected sex before the age of 16. Males with earlier onset of puberty were more likely to report fighting and aggressive responses to emotional upset during early adolescence; females were more likely to report being bullied and taking more time off school. It must be noted that for both sexes earlier pubertal onset was associated with poorer parental socioeconomic status. Similarly, Glynn and others (2010) found among young people in Malawi that earlier age at menarche was strongly associated with earlier sexual debut and marriage and lower schooling levels. They also found that the proportion of women who completed primary school was much lower among women who had experienced menarche at earlier ages.

Hormones, Mood, and Neurochemistry

Risk preferences, judgment, and decisions are affected by steroids (hormones) such as testosterone and cortisol. These hormones are associated with stress, euphoria, and fear.[10] Experimental studies have shown that high levels of testosterone increase the odds of health risk behavior (Booth, Johnson, and Granger 1999). Those who have a greater inclination to sensation-seeking tend to have higher levels of testosterone than others (Campbell and others 2010). Sensation seekers also tend to have low levels of monoamine oxidase, an enzyme that regulates serotonin, which in turn regulates mood. People with low monoamine oxidase levels tend to smoke and drink more than others and are more likely to have a criminal record (Drichoutis and Nayga 2012).

Risk preferences are sensitive to current metabolic state (Symmonds and others 2010). This is partly a matter of framing (Berns, Laibson, and Loewenstein 2007; Laibson 2001), but it is also a consequence of the presence of certain hormones during different states. Individuals became more risk-averse after a meal, as the secretion of a hormone that signals hunger falls. The impact depends both on baseline characteristics and on expectations. A smaller-than-expected meal is correlated with greater risk-seeking. As the suppression of this hormone is reduced in obesity, food consumption has a smaller effect on risk aversion (Symmonds and others 2010). This may explain why obese people have a harder time resisting food than others (Nasser, Gluck, and Geliebter 2004; Nederkoorn and others 2006).

One experimental study has shown that although women are generally more risk-averse and careful than men, women who were menstruating at the time of the experiment were more predisposed to display Allais' paradox, which might be stated in this case as miscalculating the significance of large events with small probabilities (Eckel and Grossman 2008). Experiments have shown that investors in a good mood are more risk-averse (Isen, Nygren, and Ashby 1988); anxiety and fear tends to make them even more so, choosing gambles with low-risk payoffs. Sadness makes people prone to choose high-risk gambles, whereas anger tends to make people irrationally optimistic, careless, impatient, and willing to engage in riskier gambles (Lerner and Keltner 2000, 2001), partly because it alters perceptions of control, responsibility, and certainty (Lerner and Tiedens 2006). In a well-known set of experiments (Ariely and Loewenstein 2006), subjects who would under normal ("cool") conditions exhibit normal risk aversion are induced to behave irrationally and to express a willingness to engage in high-risk or morally questionable behavior once in a state of sexual arousal (the "hot" condition). Moreover, individuals significantly overestimate their ability to remain cool and to control their behavior when aroused.

The links among mood, hormones, and risk are especially important during adolescence, at which time the body rapidly increases the production of sex hormones that impel adolescents toward thrill seeking (Barbalat and others 2010). Subsequent development provides the tools to regulate hormone secretion as well as the judgment to control the impulses that they engender. However, excessive exposure to stress, or the inability to regulate stress hormones, can also impede judgment or promote sensation-seeking (Almenberg 2009; Coates, Gurnell, and Sarnyai 2010; Stanton and others 2011).

Conclusion

This chapter has shown that decision making with respect to engagement in risky health behaviors is a complex function of many factors. The perceived cost associated with these behaviors depends on prices, information, and subjective beliefs. Individuals' valuation of their well-being in the future, which they consider to put at risk, can depend on their education, wealth, and competing health risks. Social norms and composition of social networks can alter the present benefit from these behaviors. Individuals, moreover, are not only different in the costs and benefits they face but also in the way in which they consider the trade-off between the costs and benefits. For example, individual characteristics such as impatience and lack of self-control make them more present-biased and increase their propensity to take risks. There is also evidence that better educated individuals are more likely to reduce risk-taking when exposed to information about the adverse consequences of certain behaviors.

A great deal of public health efforts aim to minimize the welfare loss and the burden on the public funds arising from poor health or premature death. Many of these efforts fail, most are only weakly effective. This failure stems partly from a misunderstanding of motives and drivers of behaviors, and the factors that condition responses to external stimuli. Addicts will respond differently from non-addicts; adolescents will respond differently from non-adolescents. Choices depend partly on prior experiences and expectations. Understanding this heterogeneity has the possibility to greatly enhance the effectiveness of investments to enhance long-term well-being and health in particular.

Notes

1. Sander (1995a, 1995b) concludes that schooling reduces the odds that both men and women will smoke and increases the odds that individuals above age

25 will quit smoking. De Walque (2007a) finds that education reduces the likelihood of men to smoke and increases the likelihood of quitting among those who have initiated smoking. Currie and Moretti (2003) find that education decreases smoking among pregnant women; smoking can harm the health of the unborn child as well as the health of the mother.

2. Other recent studies not covered due to lack of space are Clark and Royer (2010) and Kemptner, Jürges, and Reinhold (2011), who exploit changes in compulsory schooling laws in Britain and Germany, respectively, to estimate the causal effect of schooling on a range of health-related behaviors and outcomes.
3. Jukes, Simmons, and Bundy (2008) and Hargreaves and Glynn (2002) review the literature on the relationship between education and HIV infection.
4. http://www.cdc.gov/hiv/policies/law/risk.html.
5. See, for example, Chaloupka and Warner (2000), Gallett (2007), Gallet and List (2003), Grossman (2005), and Wagenaar, Salois, and Komro (2009). Cawley and Ruhm (2011) provide a detailed review of this literature.
6. Most of the literature focused on investments in education. For example, Jayachandran and Lleras-Muney (2009) find that increases in the life expectancy of girls increased investments in their education. Fortson (2011) shows that investments in education declined in areas with high levels of HIV.
7. These two competing systems are also referred to as "passions" and "interests" (Hirschman 1977), or "automatic" and "reflective" (Thaler and Sunstein 2009).
8. In the 1990s, the "Moving to Opportunity" program in five U.S. cities provided housing vouchers and assistance to approximately 4,600 families in high-poverty public housing; the families could use the vouchers to find housing in other neighborhoods (Kling and Liebman 2004).
9. Specifically, the presence of the 7-repeat allele of the DRD4 gene that regulates dopamine uptake (Dreber and others 2010).
10. Loewenstein's (2000) "visceral factors."

References

Almenberg, A. D. 2009. "Determinants of Economic Preferences." Unpublished PhD Thesis, Stockholm School of Economics, Stockholm.

Ariely, D., and G. Loewenstein. 2006. "The Heat of the Moment: The Effect of Sexual Arousal on Sexual Decision Making." *Journal of Behavioral Decision Making* 19 (2): 87–98.

Auld, M. C. 2003. "Choices, Beliefs, and Infectious Disease Dynamics." *Journal of Health Economics* 22 (3): 361–77.

Banerjee, A., and S. Mullainathan. 2010. "The Shape of Temptation: Implications for the Economic Lives of the Poor." Working Paper 15973, National Bureau of Economic Research, Cambridge, MA.

Barbalat, G., P. Domenech, M. Vernet, and P. Fourneret. 2010. "Approche neuroéconomique de la prise de risque à l'adolescence." *Encephale* 36 (2): 147–54.

Barrington, Clare, Carl Latkin, Michael D. Sweat, Luis Moreno, Jonathan Ellen, and Deanna Kerrigan. 2009. "Talking the Talk, Walking the Walk: Social Network

Norms, Communication Patterns, and Condom Use Among the Male Partners of Female Sex Workers in La Romana, Dominican Republic." *Social Science & Medicine* 68 (11): 2037–44.

Baumeister, R. F., T. F. Heatherton, and D. M. Tice. 1994. *Losing Control: How and Why People Fail at Self-Regulation.* San Diego, CA: Academic Press.

Becker, G. S. 1993. *Human Capital: A Theoretical and Empirical Analysis, with Special Reference to Education.* Chicago: University of Chicago Press.

Becker, Gary S., and Kevin M. Murphy. 1988. "A Theory of Rational Addiction." *Journal of Political Economy* 96 (4): 675–700.

Beegle, Kathleen, and Damien de Walque. 2009. "Demographic and Socioeconomic Patterns of HIV/AIDS Prevalence in Africa." Policy Research Working Paper 5076, World Bank, Washington, DC.

Ben Zion, I. Z., R. Tessler, L. Cohen, E. Lerer, Y. Raz, R. Bachner-Melman, I. Gritsenko, L. Nemanov, A. H. Zohar, R. H. Belmaker, J. Benjamin, and R. P. Ebstein. 2006. "Polymorphisms in the Dopamine D4 Receptor Gene (DRD4) Contribute to Individual Differences in Human Sexual Behavior: Desire, Arousal, and Sexual Function." *Molecular Psychiatry* 11 (8): 782–86.

Berns, G. S., D. Laibson, and G. Loewenstein. 2007. "Intertemporal Choice—Toward an Integrative Framework." *Trends in Cognitive Science* 11 (11): 482–88.

Betancourt, T. S., R. T. Brennan, J. Rubin-Smith, G. M. Fitzmaurice, and S. E. Gilman. 2010. "Sierra Leone's Former Child Soldiers: A Longitudinal Study of Risk, Protective Factors, and Mental Health." *Journal of the American Academy of Child and Adolescent Psychiatry* 49 (6): 606–15.

Bishai, David M. 2001. "Lifecycle Changes in the Rate of Time Preference: Testing the Theory of Endogenous Preferences and Its Relevance to Adolescent Substance Use." In *Economic Analysis of Substance Use and Abuse: The Experience of Developed Countries and Lessons for Developing Countries,* edited by M. Grossman and C.-R. Hsieh, 155–77. London: Edward Elgar Press.

———. 2004. "Does Time Preference Change with Age?" *Journal of Popular Economics* 17: 583–602.

Booth, A., D. R. Johnson, and D. A. Granger. 1999. "Testosterone and Men's Health." *Journal of Behavioral Medicine* 22 (1): 1–19.

Bremner, J. D. 2005. "Effects of Traumatic Stress on Brain Structure and Function: Relevance to Early Responses to Trauma." *Journal of Trauma Dissociation* 6 (2): 51–68.

Burke, M., E. Gong, and K. Jones. 2012. "Income Shocks and HIV in Sub-Saharan Africa." International Food Policy Research Institute, Washington, DC.

Campbell, B. C., A. Dreber, C. L. Apicella, D. T. Eisenberg, P. B. Gray, A. C. Little, J. R. Garcia, R. S. Zamore, and J. K. Lum. 2010. "Testosterone Exposure, Dopaminergic Reward, and Sensation-Seeking in Young Men." *Physiology & Behavior* 99: 451–56.

Cardoso, Ana Rute, and Dorte Verner. 2008. "Youth Risk-Taking Behavior in Brazil: Drug Use and Teenage Pregnancy." Working Paper 4548, World Bank, Washington, DC.

Carpenter, Jeffrey P., Justin R. Garcia, and J. Koji Lum. 2011. "Dopamine Receptor Genes Predict Risk Preferences, Time Preferences, and Related Economic Choices." *Journal of Risk Uncertainty* 42: 233–61.

Casey, B. J., L. H. Somerville, I. H. Gotlib, O. Ayduk, N. T. Franklin, M. K. Askren, J. Jonides, M. G. Berman, N. L. Wilson, T. Teslovich, G. Glover, V. Zayas, W. Mischel, and Y. Shoda. 2011. "Behavioral and Neural Correlates of Delay of Gratification 40 Years Later." *Proceedings of the National Academy of Sciences* 108 (36): 14998–5003.

Cawley, J., and C. Ruhm. 2011. "The Economics of Risky Health Behaviors." In *Handbook of Health Economics*, vol. 2, edited by Pedro Pita Barros, Tom McGuire, and Mark Pauly, 95–199. New York: Elsevier.

Centers for Disease Control and Prevention. 1993. "Mortality Trends for Selected Smoking-Related Cancers and Breast Cancer—United States, 1950–1990." *Morbidity and Mortality Weekly Report* 42 (44): 857–63.

Chaloupka, F. J., and K. E. Warner. 2000. "The Economics of Smoking." In *Handbook of Health Economics*, vol. 1, edited by A. J. Culyer and J. P. Newhouse, 1539–627. New York: Elsevier.

Chesson, Harrell W., Jami S. Leichliter, Gregory D. Zimet, Susan L. Rosenthal, David I. Bernstein, and Kenneth H. Fife. 2006. "Discount Rates and Risky Sexual Behaviors Among Teenagers and Young Adults." *Journal of Risk Uncertainty* 32: 217–30. doi: 10.1007/s11166-006-9520-1.

Christakis, Nicholas A., and James H. Fowler. 2007. "The Spread of Obesity in a Large Social Network Over 32 Years." *New England Journal of Medicine* 357: 370–79.

———. 2008. "The Collective Dynamics of Smoking in a Large Social Network." *New England Journal of Medicine* 358: 2249–58.

Cialdini, Robert B., and Melanie R. Trost. 1998. "Social Influence: Social Norms, Conformity and Compliance." In *The Handbook of Social Psychology*, 4th edition, edited by Daniel Gilbert, Susan Fiske, and Gardner Lindzey. New York: McGraw Hill.

Clark, D., and H. Royer. 2010. "The Effect of Education on Adult Health and Mortality: Evidence from Britain." Working Paper 16013, National Bureau of Economic Research, Cambridge, MA.

Coates, John M., Mark Gurnell, and Zoltan Sarnyai. 2010. "From Molecule to Market: Steroid Hormones and Financial Risk-Taking." *Philosophical Transactions of the Royal Society of Biological Sciences* 365: 331–43.

Crepaz, N., T. A. Hart, and G. Marks. 2004. "Highly Active Antiretroviral Therapy and Sexual Risk Behavior." *Journal of the American Medical Association* 292 (2): 224–36.

Currie, J., and E. Moretti. 2003. "Mother's Education and the Intergenerational Transmission of Human Capital: Evidence from College Openings." *Quarterly Journal of Economics* 118 (4): 1495–532.

Delavande, A., and H. P. Kohler. 2012. "The Impact of HIV Testing on Subjective Expectations and Risky Behavior in Malawi." *Demography* 49 (3): 1011–36.

De Paula, A., G. Shapira, and P. Todd. Forthcoming. "How Beliefs About HIV Status Affect Risky Behaviors: Evidence from Malawi." *Journal of Applied Econometrics*.

de Walque, D. 2007a. "Does Education Affect Smoking Behaviors?: Evidence Using the Vietnam Draft as an Instrument for College Education." *Journal of Health Economics* 26 (5): 877–95.

———. 2007b. "How Does the Impact of an HIV/AIDS Information Campaign Vary With Educational Attainment? Evidence from Rural Uganda." *Journal of Development Economics* 84 (2): 686–714.

———. 2009. "Does Education Affect HIV status? Evidence from Five African Countries." *The World Bank Economic Review*, 23 (2), 209–33.

———. 2010. "Education, Information and Smoking Decisions: Evidence from Smoking Histories in the United States, 1940–2000." *Journal of Human Resources* 45 (3): 682–717.

de Walque, D., and R. Kline. 2011. "The Relationship Between HIV Infection and Education: An Analysis of Six Sub-Saharan African Countries." In *The Socioeconomic Dimensions of HIV/AIDS in Africa*, edited by David E. Sahn, 110–33. Ithaca, NY: Cornell University Press.

de Walque, D., H. Kazianga, and M. Over. 2012. "Antiretroviral Therapy Awareness and Risky Sexual Behaviors: Evidence from Mozambique." *Economic Development and Cultural Change* 61 (1): 97–126.

Dinkelman, T., D. Lam, and M. Leibbrandt. 2007. "Household and Community Income, Economic Shocks, and Risky Sexual Behavior of Young Adults: Evidence from the Cape Area Panel Study 2002 and 2005." *AIDS* 21 (S7): S49.

———. 2008."Linking Poverty and Income Shocks to Risky Sexual Behaviour: Evidence From a Panel Study of Young Adults in Cape Town." *South African Journal of Economics* 76: S52–74.

Dow, W. H., T. J. Philipson, and X. Sala-i-Martin. 1999. "Longevity Complementarities Under Competing Risks." *American Economic Review* 1358–71.

Downing, J., and M. A. Bellis. 2009. "Early Pubertal Onset and Its Relationship with Sexual Risk Taking, Substance Use, and Anti-Social Behaviour: A Preliminary Cross-Sectional Study." *BMC Public Health* 9 (446).

Dreber, Anna, David G. Rand, Justin R. Garcia, Nils Wernerfelt, J. Koji Lum, and Richard Zeckhauser. 2010. "Dopamine and Risk Preferences in Different Domains." Harvard Kennedy School Working Paper RWP10-012, Harvard University, Cambridge, MA.

Drichoutis, Andreas, and Rodolfo Nayga. 2012. "Do Risk and Time Preferences Have Biological Roots?" MPRA Paper 37320.

Eckel, C. C., and P. J. Grossman. 2008. "Men, Women, and Risk Aversion: Experimental Evidence." In *Handbook of Experimental Economics Results*, edited by C. R. Plott and V. L. Smith, 106–73. New York: Elsevier.

Ethier, Kathleen A., Trace S. Kershaw, Jessica B. Lewis, Stephanie Milan, Linda M. Niccolai, and Jeannette R. Ickovics. 2006. "Self-Esteem, Emotional Distress, and Sexual Behavior Among Adolescent Females: Inter-Relationships and Temporal Effects." *Journal of Adolescent Health* 38: 268–74.

Falk, Armin. 2012. "Preferences and Personality: Heterogeneity, Determinants, and Formation." Presentation to Louis-André Gérard-Varet Conference in Public Economics, Marseille, June.

Fareri, D. S., L. N. Martin, and M. R. Delgado. 2008. "Reward-Related Processing in the Human Brain: Developmental Considerations." *Development and Psychopathology* 20 (4): 1191–211.

Farrell, P., and V. R. Fuchs. 1982. "Schooling and Health: The Cigarette Connection." *Journal of Health Economics* 1 (3): 217–30.

Fehr, Ernst. 2009. "Social Preferences and the Brain." In *Neuroeconomics: Decision Making and the Brain*, edited by Paul W. Glimcher, Ernst Fehr, Colin Camerer, and Russell Alan Poldrack. London: Elsevier.

Felitti, V. J., and R. F. Anda. 2005. "The Adverse Childhood Experiences (ACE) Study." Centers for Disease Control and Prevention and Kaiser Permanente, Atlanta, GA.

Fortson, J. G. 2008. "The Gradient in Sub-Saharan Africa: Socioeconomic Status and HIV/AIDS. *Demograph* 45 (2): 303–22.

———. 2011. "Mortality Risk and Human Capital Investment: The Impact of HIV/AIDS in Sub-Saharan Africa." *Review of Economics and Statistics* 93 (1): 1–15.

Frumence, Gasto, Malin Eriksson, Lennarth Nystrom, Japhet Killewo, and Maria Emmelin. 2011. "Exploring the Role of Cognitive and Structural Forms of Social Capital in HIV/AIDS Trends in the Kagera Region of Tanzania: A Grounded Theory Study." *African Journal of AIDS Research* 10 (1): 1–13.

Gallet, C. A. 2007. "The Demand for Alcohol: A Meta-Analysis of Elasticities." *Australian Journal of Agricultural and Resource Economics* 51 (2): 121–35.

Gallet, C. A., and J. A. List. 2003. "Cigarette Demand: A Meta-Analysis of Elasticities." *Health Economics* 12 (10): 821–35.

Gardner, Margo, and Laurence Steinberg. 2005. "Peer Influence on Risk Taking, Risk Preference, and Risky Decision Making in Adolescence and Adulthood: An Experimental Study." *Developmental Psychology* 41 (4): 625–35.

Gertler, P., M. Shah, and S. M. Bertozzi. 2005. "Risky Business: The Market for Unprotected Commercial Sex." *Journal of Political Economy* 113 (3): 518–50.

Gibney, Laura, Nazmus Saquib, and Jesse Metzger. 2003. "Behavioral Risk Factors for STD/HIV Transmission in Bangladesh's Trucking Industry." *Social Science & Medicine* 56 (7): 1411–24.

Giedd, J. N. 2008. "The Teen Brain: Insights from Neuroimaging." *Journal of Adolescent Health* 4 (4): 335–43.

Gillespie, S., S. Kadiyala, and R. Greener. 2007. "Is Poverty or Wealth Driving HIV Transmission?" *AIDS* 21: S5–16.

Glynn, J.R., N. Kayuni, S. Floyd, E. Banda, M. Francis-Chizororo, Clare Tanton, Anna Molesworth, Joanne Hemmings, Amelia Crampton, and Neil French. 2010. "Age at Menarche, Schooling, and Sexual Debut in Northern Malawi." *PLoS ONE* 5 (12): e15334.

Gong, E. 2011. "HIV Testing and Risky Sexual Behavior." Working Paper 1101, College of Economics, Middlebury College, Middlebury, VT.

Grossman, M. 1972. "On the Concept of Health Capital and the Demand for Health." *The Journal of Political Economy* 80 (2): 223–55.

———. 2005. "Individual Behaviours and Substance Use: The Role of Price." *Advances in Health Economics and Health Services Research* 16: 15–39.

Hargreaves, J. R., and J. R. Glynn. 2002. "Educational Attainment and HIV-1 Infection in Developing Countries: A Systematic Review." *Tropical Medicine & International Health* 7 (6): 489–98.

Hirschman, Albert O. 1977. *The Passions and the Interests: Political Arguments for Capitalism before Its Triumph*. Princeton, NJ: Princeton University Press.

Huebner, David M., Torsten B. Neilands, Gregory M. Rebchook, and Susan M. Kegeles. 2011. "Sorting Through Chickens and Eggs: A Longitudinal Examination of the Associations Between Attitudes, Norms, and Sexual Risk Behavior." *Health Psychology* 30 (1): 110–18.

Iorio, D., and R. Santaeulalia-Llopis. 2011. "Education, HIV Status, and Risky Sexual Behavior: How Much Does the Stage of the HIV Epidemic Matter?" Manuscript, Washington University, St. Louis, Missouri.

Isen, A. M., T. E. Nygren, and F. G. Ashby. 1988. "Influence of Positive Affect on the Subjective Utility of Gains and Losses: It Is Just Not Worth the Risk." *Journal of Personality and Social Psychology* 55: 710–17.

Jayachandran, S., and A. Lleras-Muney. 2009. "Life Expectancy and Human Capital Investments: Evidence from Maternal Mortality Declines." *Quarterly Journal of Economics* 124 (1): 349–97.

Jensen, R., and A. Lleras-Muney. 2012. "Does Staying in School (and Not Working) Prevent Teen Smoking and Drinking?" *Journal of Health Economics* 31 (4): 644–75.

Jha, Prabhat, Frank J. Chaloupka, James Moore, Vendhan Gajalakshmi, Prakash C. Gupta, Richard Peck, Samira Asma, and Witold Zatonski. 2006. "Tobacco Addiction." In *Disease Control Priorities in Developing Countries,* 2nd edition, edited by Dean T. Jamison, Joel G. Breman, Anthony R. Measham, and others 869–85. New York: Oxford University Press and the World Bank.

Jha, P., L. Vaz, F. Plummer, N. Nagelkerke, B. Willbond, E. Ngugi, S. Moses, G. John, R. Nduati, K. MacDonald, and S. Berkley. 2001. "The Evidence Base for Interventions To Prevent HIV iIfection in Low- and Middle-Income Countries." Working Paper Series WG 5, Commission on Macroeconomics and Health, Geneva.

Joseph, Natalie Pierre, Marilyn Augustyn, Howard Cabral, and Deborah A. Frank. 2006. "Preadolescents' Report of Exposure to Violence: Association with Friends' and Own Substance Use." *Journal of Adolescent Health* 38: 669–74.

Jukes, M., S. Simmons, and D. Bundy. 2008. "Education and Vulnerability: The Role of Schools in Protecting Young Women and Girls From HIV in Southern Africa." *AIDS* 22: S41–56.

Juma, M., J. Alaii, L. K. Bartholomew, L. Askew, and B. den Borne. 2013. "Risky Sexual Behavior Among Orphan and Non-Orphan Adolescents in Nyanza Province, Western Kenya." *AIDS and Behavior* 17 (3): 951.

Kemptner, D., H. Jürges, and S. Reinhold. 2011. "Changes in Compulsory Schooling and the Causal Effect of Education on Health: Evidence from Germany." *Journal of Health Economics* 30 (2): 340–54.

Kenkel, D. S. 1991. "Health Behavior, Health Knowledge, and Schooling." *Journal of Political Economy* 99 (2): 287–05.

Kincaid, D. L. 2000. "Social Networks, Ideation, and Contraceptive Behavior in Bangladesh: A Longitudinal Analysis." *Social Science & Medicine* 50: 215–31.

Kissling, Esther, Edward H. Allison, Janet A. Seeley, Steven Russell, Max Bachmann, Stanley D. Musgrave, and Simon Heck. 2005. "Fisherfolk Are Among Groups Most at Risk of HIV: Cross-Country Analysis of Prevalence and Numbers Infected." *AIDS* 19: 1939–46.

Kling, J., and J. Liebman. 2004. "Experimental Analysis of Neighborhood Effects on Youth." Working Paper Series RWP04-034, John F. Kennedy School of Government Faculty Research, Harvard University, Cambridge, MA.

Kohler, H. P., and R. L. Thornton. 2012. "Conditional Cash Transfers and HIV/AIDS Prevention: Unconditionally Promising?" *World Bank Economic Review* 26 (2): 165–90.

Laibson, D. 2001. "A Cue-Theory of Consumption." *Quarterly Journal of Economics* 116 (1): 81–119.

Latkin, C. A., S. J. Kuramoto, M. A. Davey-Rothwell, and K. E. Tobin. 2010. "Social Norms, Social Networks, and HIV Risk Behavior Among Injection Drug Users." *AIDS Behavior* 14 (5): 1159–68.

Lerner, J. S., and D. Keltner. 2000. "Beyond Valence: Toward a Model of Emotion-Specific Influences on Judgment and Choice." *Cognition and Emotion* 14: 473–93.

———. 2001. "Fear, Anger, and Risk." *Journal of Personality and Social Psychology* 81: 146–59.

Lerner, Jennifer S., and Larissa Z. Tiedens. 2006. "Portrait of the Angry Decision Maker: How Appraisal Tendencies Shape Anger's Influence on Cognition." *Journal of Behavioral Decision Making* 19: 115–37.

Liston, C., B. McEwen, and B. Casey. 2009. "Psychosocial Stress Reversibly Disrupts Prefrontal Processing and Attentional Control." *Proceedings of the National Academies of Science USA* 106: 912–17.

Loewenstein, G. 2000. "Emotions in Economic Theory and Economic Behavior." *American Economic Review* 90 (2): 426–32.

Loewenstein, G. F., and T. O'Donoghue. 2004. "Animal Spirits: Affective and Deliberative Processes in Economic Behavior." Working Paper 04-14, Center for Analytic Economics, Cornell University, Ithaca, NY.

Lurie, Mark, Abigail Harrison, David Wilkinson and Salim Abdool Karim. 1997. "Sexual Networking, Knowledge and Risk: Contextual Social Research for Confronting AIDS and STDs in Eastern and Southern Africa." *Health Transition Review* 7 (S3): 17–27.

Messiah, Antoine, Aymery Constant, Benjamin Contrand, Marie-Line Felonneau, and Emmanuel Lagarde. 2012. "Risk Compensation: A Male Phenomenon? Results From a Controlled Intervention Trial Promoting Helmet Use Among Cyclists." *American Journal of Public Health* 102 (S2): S204–06.

Middlebrooks, J. S., and N. C. Audage. 2008. "The Effects of Childhood Stress on Health Across the Lifespan." Centers for Disease Control and Prevention, National Center for Injury Prevention and Control, Atlanta.

Mischel, W., and R. Mendoza-Denton. 2003. "Harnessing Willpower and Socioemotional Intelligence To Enhance Human Agency and Potential." In *A Psychology of Human Strengths: Fundamental Questions and Future Directions for a Positive Psychology*, edited by L. G. Aspinwall and U. M. Staudinger, 245–56. Washington, DC: American Psychological Association.

Mishra, V., S. Bignami-Van Assche, R. Greener, M. Vaessen, R. Hong, P. D. Ghys, and S. Rutstein. 2007. "HIV Infection Does Not Disproportionately Affect the Poorer in Sub-Saharan Africa." *AIDS* 21: S17–28.

Mkandawire, Paul, Eric Tenkorang, and Isaa N. Luginaah. 2012. "Orphan Status and Time to First Sex among Adolescents in Northern Malawi." *AIDS and Behavior* 17 (3): 939–50.

Morgan, D., C. Mahe, B. Mayanja, J. M. Okongo, R. Lubega, and J. A. Whitworth. 2002. "HIV-1 Infection in Rural Africa: Is There a Difference in Median Time to AIDS and Survival Compared With That in Industrialized Countries?" *AIDS* 16 (4): 597–603.

Morojele, Neo K., and Judith S. Brook. 2006. "Substance Use and Multiple Victimisation Among Adolescents in South Africa." *Addictive Behaviors* 31: 1163–76.

Muraven, M., D. M. Tice, and R. F. Baumeister. 1998. "Self-Control as a Limited Resource: Regulatory Depletion Patterns." *Journal of Personality and Social Psychology* 74: 774–89.

Nasser J. A., M. E. Gluck, and A. Geliebter. 2004. "Impulsivity and Test Meal Intake in Obese Binge Eating Women." *Appetite* 43: 303–07.

Nederkoorn, C., C. Braet, Y. Van Eijs, A. Tanghe, and A. Jansen. 2006. "Why Obese Children Cannot Resist Food: The Role of impulsivity." *Eating Behaviors* 7: 315–22.

Operario D., K. Underhill, C. Chuong, and L. Cluver. 2011. "HIV Infection and Sexual Risk Behaviour Among Youth Who Have Experienced Orphanhood: Systematic Review and Meta-Analysis." *Journal of the International AIDS Society* 18 (14): 25.

Orphanides, A., and D. Zervos. 1995. "Rational Addiction with Learning and Regret." *Journal of Political Economy* 103 (4): 739–58.

Orubuloye, I. O., Pat Caldwell, and John C. Caldwell. 1993. "The Role of High-Risk Occupations in the Spread of AIDS: Truck Drivers and Itinerant Market Women in Nigeria." *International Family Planning Perspectives* 19 (2): 43–48, 71.

Oster, E. 2012. "HIV and Sexual Behavior Change: Why Not Africa?" *Journal of Health Economics* 31 (1): 35–49.

Peltzman, S. 1975. "The Effects of Automobile Safety Regulation." *Journal of Political Economy* 83 (4): 677–725.

Pharo, H., C. Sim, M. Graham, J. Gross, and H. Hayne. 2011. "Risky Business: Executive Function, Personality, and Reckless Behavior During Adolescence and Emerging Adulthood." *Behavioral Neuroscience* 125 (6): 970–88. Epub 2011 Oct 17.

Pickering, H., M. Okongo, B. Nnalusiba, K. Bwanika, and J. Whitworth. 1997. "Sexual Networks in Uganda: Casual and Commercial Sex in a Trading Town." *AIDS Care* 9 (2): 199–208.

Pronyk, P. M., T. Harpham, L. A. Morison, J. R. Hargreaves, J. C. Kim, G. Phetla, C. H. Watts, and J. D. Porter. 2008. "Is Social Capital Associated with HIV Risk in Rural South Africa?" *Social Science and Medicine* 66 (9): 1999–2010.

Rao, V., L. Gupta, M. Lokshin, and S. Jana. 2003. "Sex Workers and the Cost of Safe Sex: The Compensating Differential for Condom Use among Calcutta Prostitutes." *Journal of Development Economics* 71 (2): 585–603.

Robinson, J., and E. Yeh. 2011. "Transactional Sex as a Response to Risk in Western Kenya." *American Economic Journal: Applied Economics* 3 (1): 35–64.

———. 2012. "Risk-Coping through Sexual Networks: Evidence from Client Transfers in Kenya." *Journal of Human Resources* 47 (1): 107–45.

Romer, Daniel, Angela L. Duckworth, Sharon Sznitman, and Sunhee Park. 2010. "Can Adolescents Learn Self-Control? Delay of Gratification in the Development of Control over Risk Taking." Manuscript, University of Pennsylvania. *Prevention Science* 11(3): 319–30. doi: 10.1007/s11121-010-0171-8.

Sander, W. 1995a. "Schooling and Quitting Smoking." *Review of Economics and Statistics* 77 (1): 191–99.

———. 1995b. "Schooling and Smoking." *Economics of Education Review* 14 (1): 23–33.

Seeyave, Desiree M., Sharon Coleman, Danielle Appugliese, Robert F. Corwyn, Robert H. Bradley, Natalie S. Davidson, Niko Kaciroti, and Julie C. Lumeng. 2009. "Ability to Delay Gratification at Age 4 Years and Risk of Overweight at Age 11 Years." *Archives of Pediatric Adolescent Medicine* 163 (4): 303–08.

Selikow, Terry-Ann, Nazeema Ahmed, Alan J. Flisher, Catherine Mathews, and Wanjiru Mukoma. 2009. "'I Am Not "Umqwayito:"' A Qualitative Study of Peer Pressure and Sexual Risk Behaviour Among Young Adolescents in Cape Town, South Africa." *Scandinavian Journal of Public Health* 37: 107–12.

Shiv, Baba, and Alexander Fedorikhin. 1999. "Heart and Mind in Conflict: The Interplay of Affect and Cognition in Consumer Decision Making." *Journal of Consumer Research* 26 (3): 278–92.

Simons-Morton, Bruce G., Marie Claude Ouimet, Zhiwei Zhang, Sheila E. Klauer, Suzanne E. Lee, Jing Wang, Rusan Chen, Paul Albert, and Thomas A. Dingus. 2011. "The Effect of Passengers and Risk-Taking Friends on Risky Driving and Crashes/Near Crashes Among Novice Teenagers." *Journal of Adolescent Health* 49 (6): 587–93.

Simpson, Jeffrey A., Vladas Griskevicius, Sally i-Chun Kuo, Sooyeon Sung, and W. Andrew Collins. 2012. "Evolution, Stress, and Sensitive Periods: The Influence of Unpredictability in Early Versus Late Childhood on Sex and Risky Behavior." *Developmental Psychology* 48 (3): 674–86.

Slovic, Paul. 2000. "What Does It Mean to Know a Cumulative Risk? Adolescents' Perceptions of Short-Term and Long-Term Consequences of Smoking." *Journal of Behavioral Decision Making* 13: 259–66.

———. 2001. "Cigarette Smokers: Rational Actors or Rational Fools? In *Smoking: Risk, Perception, & Policy*, edited by P. Slovic, 97–124. Thousand Oaks, CA: Sage.

Smith, J., F. Nalagoda, M. J. Wawer, D. Serwadda, N. Sewankambo, J. Konde-Lule, T. Latalo, C. Li, and R. H. Gray. 1999. "Education Attainment as a Predictor of HIV Risk in Rural Uganda: Results From a Population-Based Study. *International Journal of STD & AIDS* 10 (7): 452–59.

Spears, D. 2010. "Economic Decision-Making in Poverty Depletes Cognitive Control." Unpublished manuscript, Princeton University, Princeton, NJ.

Stanton, Steven J., A. Mullette-Gillman O'Dhaniel, R. Edward McLaurin, Cynthia M. Kuhn, Kevin S. LaBar, Michael L. Platt, and Scott A. Huettel. 2011. "Low- and High-Testosterone Individuals Exhibit Decreased Aversion to Economic Risk." *Psychological Science* 22 (4): 447–53.

Steinberg, Laurence. 2008. "A Social Neuroscience Perspective on Adolescent Risk-Taking." *Development Review* (1): 78–106. doi:10.1016/j.dr.2007.08.002.

Stoel, R. D., E. J. C. De Geus, and D. I. Boomsma. 2006. "Genetic Analysis of Sensation Seeking with an Extended Twin Design." *Behavior Genetics* 36: 229–37.

Sutter, Matthias, Martin G. Kocher, Daniela Rützler, and Stefan T. Trautmann. 2010. "Impatience and Uncertainty: Experimental Decisions Predict Adolescents' Field Behavior." Discussion Paper No. 5404, Institute for the Study of Labor, Bonn.

Symmonds, M., J. J. Emmanuel, M. E. Drew, R. L. Batterham, and R. J. Dolan. 2010. "Metabolic State Alters Economic Decision Making under Risk in Humans." *PLoS ONE* 5 (6): e11090. doi:10.1371/journal.pone.0011090.

Thaler, R. H., and C. R. Sunstein. 2009. *Nudge: Improving Decisions About Health, Wealth, and Happiness*. New York: Penguin Books.

Thurman, T. R., L. Brown, L. Richter, P. Maharaj, and R. Magnani. 2006. "Sexual Risk Behavior Among South African Adolescents: Is Orphan Status a Factor?" *AIDS and Behavior* 10 (6): 627–35.

Tsukayama, Eli, Angela Lee Duckworth, and Betty Kim. n.d. "Resisting Everything Except Temptation: Evidence for Domain-Specific and Domain-General Aspects of Impulsive Behavior." Manuscript, University of Pennsylvania.

Varga, C. A. 2001. "Coping with HIV/AIDS in Durban's Commercial Sex Industry." *AIDS Care* 13 (3): 351–65.

Voors, Maarten J., Eleonora E. M. Nillesen, Philip Verwimp, Erwin H. Bulte, Robert Lensink, and Daan P. Van Soest. 2012. "Violent Conflict and Behavior: A Field Experiment in Burundi." *American Economic Review* 102 (2): 941–64.

Vrolix, Klara. 2006. "Behavioural Adaptation, Risk Compensation, Risk Homeostasis, and Moral Hazard in Traffic Safety." Universiteit Hasselt, Steunpunt Verkeersveiligheid.

Vuchinich, Rudy E., and Cathy A. Simpson. 1998. "Hyperbolic Temporal Discounting in Social Drinkers and Problem Drinkers." *Experimental and Clinical Psychopharmacology* 6: 1–14.

Wagenaar, A. C., M. J. Salois, and K. A. Komro. 2009. "Effects of Beverage Alcohol Price and Tax Levels on Drinking: A Meta-Analysis of 1003 Estimates from 112 Studies." *Addiction* 104 (2): 179–90.

Wilde, Gerald J. S. 2002. "Does Risk Homoeostasis Theory Have Implications for Road Safety?" *British Medical Journal* 324: 1149–52.

Wilson, N. 2012. "Economic Booms and Risky Sexual Behavior: Evidence from Zambian Copper Mining Cities." *Journal of Health Economics* 31 (6): 797–812.

Wittmann, M., and M. P. Paulus. 2007. "Decision Making, Impulsivity, and Time Perception." *Trends in Cognitive Science* 12 (1): 7–12.

Yang, Cui, Carl A. Latkin, Peng Liu, Kenrad E. Nelson, Cunlin Wang, and Rongsheng Luan. 2010. "A Qualitative Study on Commercial Sex Behaviors Among Male Clients in Sichuan Province, China." *AIDS Care* 22 (2): 246–52.

Zyphur, Michael J., Jayanth Narayanan, Richard D. Arvey, and Gordon J. Alexander. 2009. "The Genetics of Economic Risk Preferences." *Journal of Behavioral Decision Making* 22 (4): 367–77.

3

The Consequences of Risky Behaviors

Alaka Holla

Introduction

Regardless of what drives people to engage in behaviors like smoking, unhealthy eating, or risky sex, the consequences of these behaviors are more easily observable. These behaviors typically lead to diseases or injuries that require expensive treatment over the long run and that interfere with productivity. In the absence of well-developed markets for health and disability insurance in many low-income countries, individuals will face limited options for arresting the declines in their own health and for smoothing their consumption once the risks associated with these behaviors have been realized. These behaviors and their associated illnesses also generate spillovers beyond individuals and often adversely affect their children, family members, and coworkers. To the extent that health systems must absorb some of the costs of treatment and that the disease consequences of these behaviors prematurely remove a nontrivial number of people from the labor force, these spillovers can even extend to the larger society.

This chapter attempts to quantify the impacts of risky behaviors by focusing on three types of consequences:

- Those that accrue to the individual engaging in the risky behavior
- Those that spill over to the individual's peers—people in the same household or coworkers

- Those that society must bear either through public health expenditures or through a decline in aggregate productivity that results from premature exits from the labor force.

A great deal of research in the fields of public health and medicine has focused on quantifying these kinds of effects, although data constraints have limited most studies to high-income countries. Most of the people afflicted with the chronic diseases that result from these risky behaviors, however, live in low-income countries, where these behaviors are in fact becoming the leading risk factors for mortality and morbidity. In high-income countries, the resulting diseases mostly affect older people, but in low-income settings, these illnesses tend to affect the working-age population, leading not only to longer periods of elevated health care costs but also to greater losses in productivity. From the perspective of policy, it is important to quantify these impacts. If the implied welfare declines experienced by individuals are large, as well as the externalities they generate, then market failures like inadequate insurance markets or externalities to third parties make a clear case for governments or other parties interested in social welfare to intervene and decrease the frequency of these behaviors.

Individual Consequences

Studies of these impacts on life expectancy, health expenditures, and productivity typically make use of household surveys and data from health facilities to estimate how much of a specific disease's prevalence can be explained by a specific risk factor—for example, how much of the observed prevalence of cardiovascular disease can be attributed to smoking?

To do this estimation, much of the public health and epidemiological literatures try to calculate the *population attributable risk*—that is, the proportion of risk of a disease in a population attributable to a specific factor. This is meant to capture the reduction in disease incidence that would be observed if no one in the population engaged in the risky behavior, compared to current behavior patterns. While a zero prevalence might be an unrealistic counterfactual, this calculation depends on the relative risk of dying from or contracting a disease, which is calculated by comparing mortality or disease risks of individuals who engage in a particular risky behavior to the corresponding risks of similar people who abstain from the behavior. For example, the risk of dying from lung cancer might be six times higher for smokers than nonsmokers. This exercise is typically done in a cohort study (where people are tracked across time, both before and after they develop a disease) or case-control study (where those who engage in the risky behavior are matched with those who do not along a number of characteristics). The population attributable risk is then calculated as the difference between the incidence of the disease as a fraction of all deaths in the overall population and the incidence of the disease as a fraction of all deaths among those who do not engage in the risky behavior.

These population attributable fractions give some indication of a risk factor's importance in explaining variation in disease, since we know that the diseases are not triggering the risky behaviors. However, we should be cautious in interpreting these estimates as capturing causal relationships between risky behaviors and disease. In 2010, the top 10 leading risk factors for disease were high blood pressure, tobacco smoking, alcohol use, household air pollution from solid fuels, diets low in fruits, high body mass index, high fasting plasma glucose, childhood underweight, ambient particulate matter pollution, and physical inactivity and low physical activity (Lim and others 2012). At least seven of these 10 risk factors can be linked to the risky behaviors examined in this volume, but some of these risk factors may be highly correlated. For example, people who engage in little physical activity are very likely going to display high body mass indexes. People could also engage in more than one risky behavior at once. For example, cardiovascular disease can be caused by smoking and obesity. Smokers can concurrently engage in a host of other behaviors that can increase their heart attack potential, such as eating one too many french fries, and obese people typically suffer from high blood sugar, high cholesterol, and high blood pressure. Unless a data set allows comparisons that hold all of these other variables constant, the estimates for the relative risk associated with these behaviors could be biased. These estimated population attributable risks often do not take this limitation into account. As a result, the estimated population attributable risks for multiple factors can sometimes sum to over 100 percent.

We must also exercise caution when interpreting studies that calculate how much money individuals must spend to treat the diseases or injuries that result from risky behavior. The costs of most treatments are higher in wealthy countries, for example, but this does not necessarily indicate that the illnesses pose a larger problem in these studies. In fact, it could very well be the case that affluent societies just have more expensive treatment options. The cost of illness, however, is typically the only metric we have available to quantify economic impacts on individuals, their peers, and society.

Smoking

Some research shows that once addicted to nicotine, individuals may experience short-term benefits from smoking, such as reductions in anxiety (Crisp and others 1999; Perkins and others 1999) or appetite suppression

(Aubin and others 2012), both of which may help poor people to deal with the stresses and budget constraints they confront daily. The vast majority of empirical studies, however, have focused on quantifying the costs associated with smoking, and these are substantial.

Costs of smoking

To get a sense of what opportunity costs this expenditure entails, we can convert the cost of cigarettes into the working time required to earn the same amount or to the number of calories that could have been purchased (table 3.1). In Kenya, for example, a smoker would have to work for nearly an hour to earn a packet of cigarettes or forgo the caloric equivalent of meals for nearly two and half days, if we assume a daily requirement of 2,000 calories (figure 3.1). In Romania and South Africa, money spent on one pack of cigarettes could purchase three to four days' worth of caloric requirements.

Some studies have further investigated the opportunity costs of smoking using data from household surveys. In the Philippines, for example, smoking tobacco accounted for 2.6 percent of monthly expenditures in households just below the poverty line in 2003, which exceeded their spending on clothing (2.6 percent), education (1.6 percent), and health (1.3 percent) (Baquilod and others 2008). For the poorest households, average monthly tobacco expenditure was more than 12 times the per capita monthly expenditure on health, eight times that for education, and five times that for clothing. If we think of this as additional income coming into the household and allocate 61 percent to food expenditures (the average percentage of total spending represented by food expenditures), then each month poor

Table 3.1 Opportunity Costs of Smoking

	Minutes of labor required to buy a packet of cigarettes	Kilograms of rice that can be purchased
Kenya	57	1.39
India	47	1.18
Romania	46	1.70
Malaysia	37	1.76
Peru	35	2.19
Mexico	35	1.59
South Africa	26	2.36
Thailand	25	1.25

Source: Data for minutes of labor required are from Eriksen, Mackay, and Ross 2012; Kilograms of rice derived from UBS 2012.

Figure 3.1 Calories That Can Be Purchased with the Cost of One Pack of Cigarettes

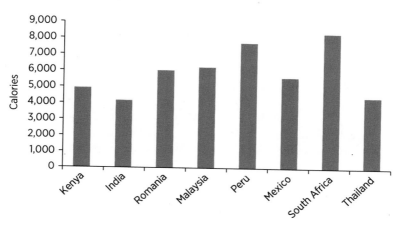

Source: Kilograms of rice are derived from UBS 2012.

Note: Calories are derived from the assumption that 100 grams of uncooked rice provides 350 calories.

households could have purchased an additional kilogram of meat or fish, 22 chicken eggs, or 53 bananas.

Disease burden of smoking

Smokers develop debilitating, often fatal, illnesses, such as cancer, cardiovascular and circulatory disease, and chronic respiratory disease.[1] The chemicals in tobacco smoke damage the lungs, blood vessels, and other tissues and keep them inflamed, disrupting the way the body can heal itself. When blood vessels thicken and narrow in this way, they make blood clots, heart attacks, and strokes more likely. When a person's airways and lungs suffer this kind of damage, the body's ability to clear the lungs and exchange oxygen becomes compromised, leading to lung diseases such as emphysema, chronic bronchitis, and pneumonia. These chemicals can also destroy a cell's ability to regulate its own growth and thereby increase the likelihood of cancers.

Not surprisingly, the Global Burden of Disease Study 2010 found that tobacco smoking (including secondhand smoke) was the second leading risk factor for the global burden of disease, accounting for nearly 6.3 million deaths in 2010. For men, it was the leading risk factor (Lim and others 2012). Nearly 80 percent of these deaths occurred in middle- and low-income countries; in China, where smoking accounts for 1.2 million deaths annually, it is the number one killer (Eriksen, Mackay, Ross 2012).

The Life Span Study (LSS) in Hiroshima and Nagasaki, Japan, was a prospective cohort study, where researchers followed respondents over time and could therefore associate baseline characteristics with future medical conditions (as opposed to associating retrospective reports of respondents' behavior with current outcomes). The LSS recorded whether respondents smoked from 1963 to 1992. One analysis estimates that among those born between 1920 and 1954 who started smoking before the age of 20, male smokers lost an average of approximately eight years of life expectancy and female smokers lost nearly 10 years, even after adjustments for potential confounders, such as education, alcohol intake, body mass index, and radiation from the atomic bombs (Sakata and others 2012).

A few studies have tried to isolate the impact of smoking from other potentially confounding risky behaviors by taking advantage of policies or factors in the environment that should trigger variation in smoking but that would have nothing to do with other aspects of smokers' behavior that could affect their health. One study in the United States, for example, tried to take advantage of the fact that the U.S. military distributed free cigarettes to overseas personnel during World War II and the Korean War (Bedard and Deschênes 2006). The study first combined census data with mortality data that lists a cause of death to find that birth cohorts with more veterans from these wars displayed higher mortality rates due to smoking-related illnesses (ischemic heart disease, lung cancer, respiratory disease) compared to cohorts with fewer veterans. For non-smoking-related conditions (colon cancer, cerebrovascular disease, and accidents and suicides), however, cohorts with more veterans had similar mortality rates to cohorts with fewer veterans.[2]

From a large consumption survey that also reports veteran status (the Current Population Survey), the study then estimates a military-induced increase in smoking of 27.6 percentage points. The study then combines these results with estimates for the population attributable fraction of smoking for lung cancer and heart disease to calculate that smoking accounted for 64–79 percent of excess mortality due to heart disease and 35–58 percent due to lung cancer. In fact, these numbers suggest that the total years of potential life lost due to smoking-induced premature death between the ages of 40 and 65 equaled the years of potential life lost due to battle deaths during World War II and the Korean War combined.

Smoking's health impact, however, is not limited to noncommunicable diseases. It has also emerged as a significant risk factor for tuberculosis in a recent systematic review of 50 studies (WHO and International Union Against Tuberculosis and Lung Disease 2007). In 44 of the included studies, smoking was significantly associated with excess risk of a tuberculosis outcome (infection, disease, recurrence, or death), even in empirical specifications that adjusted for potential confounders such as alcohol use and poverty.

Smoking-related medical care

The diseases that result from smoking trigger additional expenditures on medical care. A study in Bangladesh, for example, found that households with at least one member afflicted by a tobacco-related illness (ischemic heart disease, chronic obstructive pulmonary disease (COPD), lung cancer, laryngeal cancer, oral cancer, tuberculosis, Brueger's disease, or stroke) spent 5.1 percent of their total household monthly expenditure on tobacco and 10.2 percent on treating their illnesses; however, we cannot attribute all of this health expenditure to smoking, since it is not the sole risk factor for these illnesses (WHO 2005). Data from a hospital survey, however, indicate that the population attributable fraction of smoking for these diseases was over 50 percent on average, exceeding 70 percent for the tobacco-related cancers and chronic obstructive pulmonary disease. When a member of these households had to be hospitalized for one of these conditions, out-of-pocket hospital expenditures were more than six times total monthly expenditure.

In Vietnam, even after accounting for government subsidies, the out-of-pocket expenses for each hospital admission of lung cancer, COPD, and ischemic heart disease amounted to $285 (Ross, vu Trung, and Xuan Phu 2007) or approximately 34 percent of per capita gross domestic product (GDP).

Declines in labor productivity

Finally, both smoking itself and its associated illnesses generate substantial losses in terms of labor productivity. The Vietnam study (Ross and others 2007), for example, estimated a loss in individual earnings associated with a tobacco-related hospitalization equal to GDP per capita. Another study in Taiwan, China (Tsai and others 2005), used data from a survey of firms and the country's Institute for Occupational Safety and Health and an estimate of smokers' excess sick leave from a DuPont factory study to monetize the value of excess workplace absence and smoking breaks that go along with smoking. It estimates that smokers take an additional 0.9 days in sick leave and 9 days a year when you add up the time associated with smoking breaks, which was estimated by conservatively assuming that smoking employees only smoked during working hours if their company had a separate smoking room, they smoked only three cigarettes in the workplace, and it took six minutes to smoke one cigarette. While other factors could lie behind the excess absence from work (for example, if the smokers are also more likely to be battling alcoholism or depression at the same time), the losses from smoking breaks far outweigh the losses from absence.

Obesity

As with smoking, being overweight or obese leads to chronic illnesses that lower life expectancy, require substantial health care expenditures, and depress labor productivity. Obese people are much more likely to suffer from cardiovascular problems (hypertension, stroke, and coronary heart disease), diabetes, gallbladder disease, osteoarthritis, and certain types of cancers. The insulin hormone helps to regulate glucose levels in the blood, but having too many fat cells can lead to insulin resistance, which in turn leads to diabetes. Excess fat cells also lie behind leptin resistance, which can dull signals of satiation after eating and thus lead to even more overeating.

Disease burden of obesity

According to the Global Burden of Disease 2010 study, 11 of the top 20 risk factors for burden of disease are related to diet or physical inactivity (Lim and others 2012).[3] Cardiovascular disease is the leading cause of death in all World Bank regions except Sub-Saharan Africa, where it trails HIV/AIDS, although among people older than 30 years, it is the leading cause of death in Sub-Saharan Africa as well (Gaziano 2005). By 2000, most people with diabetes lived in a low-income country; in Asian countries, the disease appears to affect people at lower levels of obesity and at younger ages. The prevalence of obesity in India and Thailand, for example, does not amount to even half of the level observed in the United States, yet both countries exhibit diabetes prevalence that is nearly 50 percent higher (Yoon and others 2006).

There has been much less research, however, isolating the impact of diet and physical activity alone on these chronic diseases, partly because of measurement issues and partly because a number of confounding unhealthy behaviors can dampen any association between obesity and mortality that we might find in the data. While most studies use body mass index to categorize people as normal, overweight, and obese, there is evidence that weight gain independent of body mass index and the specific distribution of fat (in particular, abdominal fat) are also important risk factors. To quantify the relative importance of these factors, a case-control study matched close to 12,500 cases of a first myocardial infarction (heart attack) in 262 hospitals across 52 countries with people of the same gender and age who happened to be in the health center at the same time (for example, relatives of patients from noncardiac wards or attendants of other cardiac patients). The increased risk of a heart attack associated with body mass index diminished after an adjustment for waist-to-hip ratios, and it disappeared after adjustment for other risk factors, such as smoking or alcohol use (Yusuf and others 2005).[4] The population attributable risk of a heart attack associated with being in the top two quintiles of body mass index was 7.7 percent, whereas it reached 24.3 percent for being in the top two quintiles of waist-to-hip ratio.

In China, nearly 62 percent of all deaths in urban China in 2000 have been attributed to diet-related chronic diseases (Popkin 2008) with methods that combine information on relative risks from studies from around the world (primarily high-income countries) and prevalence of obesity and chronic diseases in China.

The costs of obesity-related medical care

The economic burden of treating these chronic conditions is particularly heavy in low-income countries, where people become ill at earlier ages. Nearly 80 percent of all cardiovascular-related deaths occur when people are over the age of 60 in high-income countries, in contrast to 42 percent in low- and middle-income countries (Gaziano 2007).

In Colombia, Nicaragua, and Peru, for example, the fraction of household expenditures financed through out-of-pocket payments for health services in households with at least one member afflicted by a chronic disease was nearly twice as high as in households with no members affected by a chronic disease (Bonilla-Chacín 2012). Among diabetic patients of a regional hospital in Kilimanjaro, Tanzania, the cost of their first visit and a month's supply of insulin amounted to 25 percent of the minimum wage (Neuhann and others 2002).

Low-income countries generally spend considerably less per patient on managing diabetes (map 3.1). Moreover, the costs of treatment are prohibitively high in all countries when we benchmark them against per capita health expenditures. Table 3.2 lists the ratio of average diabetes-related expenditures per diabetic patient to health expenditures per capita for

Map 3.1 Annual Per-Patient Spending for Diabetes Management

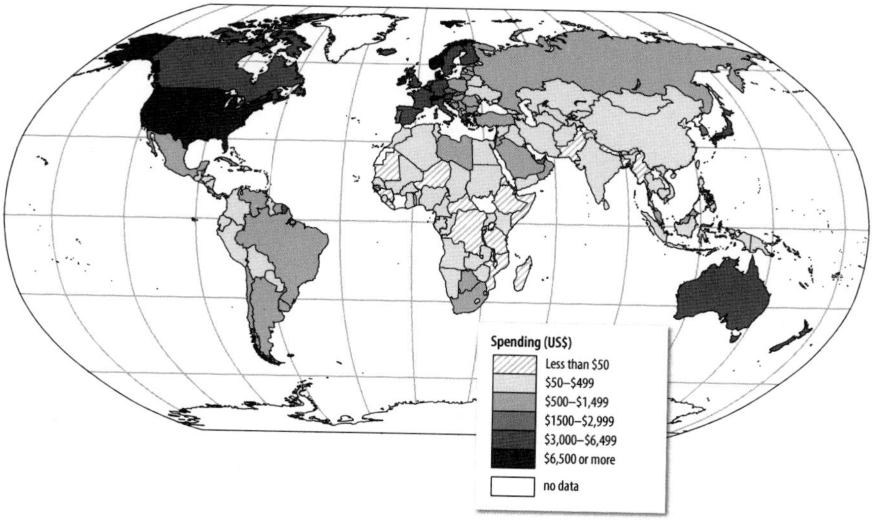

Spending (US$)

- Less than $50
- $50–$499
- $500–$1,499
- $1500–$2,999
- $3,000–$6,499
- $6,500 or more
- no data

Source: Diabetes Atlas, International Diabetes Foundation.

Table 3.2 Diabetes Expenditure in 2012

	Diabetes prevalence (percent)	Average diabetes-related expenditure per person with diabetes (US$)	Diabetes-related expenditure as a percentage of GDP/capita	Diabetes-related expenditure as a percentage of health expenditure/capita
Madagascar	5.1	38	9%	237%
Zambia	5.1	125	10%	171%
Togo	5.2	63	12%	155%
São Tomé and Príncipe	5.5	162	13%	180%
Malawi	5.6	31	9%	122%
Vietnam	5.8	118	10%	142%
Cameroon	6.2	109	10%	178%
Tajikistan	6.3	61	7%	124%
Kyrgyz Republic	6.3	79	9%	148%
Uzbekistan	6.4	80	6%	97%
Papua New Guinea	6.5	70	5%	142%
Haiti	6.7	68	10%	148%
Bolivia	6.9	125	6%	129%
Bangladesh	7.1	28	4%	121%
Afghanistan	7.6	81	18%	214%
Pakistan	7.9	36	3%	163%
Comoros	8.4	46	6%	137%
India	9.0	68	5%	125%
Sudan	9.1	151	10%	179%
Yemen, Rep.	9.2	121	9%	191%
Nicaragua	11.6	172	12%	166%
Solomon Islands	15.3	107	8%	100%
Kiribati	25.5	232	16%	145%

Source: Data on diabetes prevalence and spending are from the Diabetes Atlas, International Diabetes Foundation; data on per capita GDP and health expenditures come from the World Development Indicators.

countries with prevalence rates higher than 5 percent and GDP per capita less than US$2,000 in 2010. In Madagascar, for example, the US$38 average annual cost of treating a diabetic patient, which likely reflects the dearth of appropriate treatment options in the country rather than low prices of necessary medication, amounts to 9 percent of GDP per capita and 240 percent of health expenditures per capita. The latter figure mixes public and private expenditures, but in most of these countries (with the exceptions of Haiti, Kiribati, Madagascar, Malawi, Papua New Guinea, Solomon Islands, and Zambia), out-of-pocket payments represent more than 85 percent of private health expenditures (WHO, Global Health Expenditure Database). Individuals (and potentially their families) must therefore bear a substantial portion of these health costs.

Declines in productivity

As with smoking, evidence suggests that these expensive diseases also reduce productivity. While establishing whether obesity is consistently associated with wages and the likelihood of employment could be informative, it might not tell us whether the condition affects a person's ability to perform. It appears there is a return to physical appearance in the labor market (Hamermesh and Biddle 1994), which could differ across countries (Prentice 2006) and socioeconomic groups (Cawley 2004). Indeed, in an audit study in Sweden, job applications with a photo manipulated to make the fictitious applicant seem obese were significantly less likely to receive callbacks for interviews than when the normal weight photos were attached to the application (Rooth 2009).

Sick leave, however, is an indicator that should give us a sense of the extent to which people cannot work, either because they have to seek health care or because they find it physically difficult to get through the work day. In a national workplace survey in the United States covering more than 10,000 men and women, obese employees were 53 percent more likely to have taken off seven or more illness-related days than non-obese employees and 74 percent more likely than colleagues classified as lean, after an adjustment for standard controls such as age, gender, smoking behavior, family income, and the length of the work week (Tucker and Friedman 1998). Obese and overweight individuals were also more likely to report deficits in their ability to perform activities of daily living, such as dressing, bathing, feeding, and getting out of a chair without assistance (Peeters and others 2003).

Risky Sex

It is easier to quantify the short-term economic benefits that often follow risky sex. For commercial sex workers, for example, there could be a premium for not using a condom. Using a panel data set that allows comparison of the different sexual encounters of a commercial sex worker, a study from Mexico finds that commercial sex workers can earn a 23 percent premium for unprotected sex if their clients request that they not use a condom, compared to the encounters when clients do not request this form of risky sex (Gertler, Shah, and Bertozzi 2005). A study in a red light district of Calcutta, India, estimates a per-encounter earnings penalty of 66 to 79 percent from condom use (Rao and others 2003).

Risky sex can offer benefits even to women who are not commercial sex workers who may engage in transactional sex to smooth consumption or obtain luxury goods. A Kenyan study among formal and informal sex workers found that 84 percent held another job and that they would increase risky sexual behavior (seeing a client by 3.1 percent, anal sex by 21.2 percent, and unprotected sex by 19.1 percent) on days when a household member fell ill (Robinson and Yeh 2011). Estimated premia were 42 Kenyan shillings (US$0.60) for unprotected sex and 77 shillings (US$1.10) for anal sex. Another Kenyan study compared the sexual encounters of the same men when they use a condom and when they do not; it found a positive association between monetary transfers and unprotected sex in informal sexual relationships. For an increase of 500 shillings (US$7.14), which is the amount of the average transfer, condom use dropped 8 percent (Luke 2006).

In an ethnographic study in rural Tanzania, researchers found that transactional sex underlies most nonmarital relationships; other than escaping poverty, motivations included acquiring beauty products, such as scented soap or lotion, often given in-kind in exchange for sex, and accumulating business capital (Wamoyi and others 2010). Women who could not get money in this way were ridiculed.

Disease burden of risky sex

These risks, however, bring substantial costs in terms of disease and death in the medium to long run, especially in poorer countries. While this chapter focuses on HIV/AIDS, risky sex also leaves individuals vulnerable to all sexually transmitted infections.[5] A meta-analysis of 25 different study populations found that the estimates of HIV transmission risks per sexual act were higher in low-income countries among samples without exposure to commercial sex. In high-income countries, estimated female-to-male and male-to-female transmission risks were 0.04 percent and 0.08 percent per act, respectively, while they were 0.36 percent and 0.30 percent in low-income countries (Boily and others 2009).

A study in Bobo Dioulasso, Burkina Faso, that measured HIV prevalence among different subgroups of the population found high prevalence of infection, even among women who did not identify themselves as commercial sex workers (Nagot and others 2002). While 6.5 percent of general female population and 57 percent of commercial sex workers who practiced out of a single location were infected, nonprofessional sellers of sex—typically food vendors and barmaids—exhibited prevalences of 37 percent and 40 percent, respectively. This was higher than among women who roamed around the city looking for clients and self-identified as commercial sex workers (29 percent); it was consistent with the higher likelihood of the nonprofessionals to engage in sex without a condom relative to the professionals. While this sample of women was certainly not randomly selected (the researchers had to rely on peers to find sufficient women in each category), it does provide strong evidence of the increased risk for disease that follows risky sex.

Given the differences in health systems and disease environments, these increased rates of infection translate into higher rates of mortality in low-income countries. In high-income countries, for example, mortality among people living with AIDS was 1.0 to 1.5 percent in 2009, whereas it was 5.7 percent in low-income countries (Haacker 2013).

The costs of risky sex–related medical care

Before infected individuals die, however, they (and their families) must spend a considerable amount of their income on treatment. One study in an area in Tanzania that had a demographic surveillance system with HIV testing compiled a set of deaths among adults ages 15 to 59. It examined differences between those who had died from AIDS and those who died from other causes (Ngalula and others 2002). Relative to other diseases, health expenditures triggered by HIV/AIDS were over 70 percent greater than for other diseases over a two-year period. Together with funeral costs, this amounted to more than 100 percent of annual household income.

Declines in employment and productivity

A cohort study on a tea estate in Kenya used administrative data from the tea company's records to estimate the impact of the disease on workers' productivity (Fox and others 2004). In particular, the AIDS patients were matched to comparison tea pluckers who worked on the same field during the same time period. Three years prior to death or retirement, there were no significant differences in the number of days plucking, nor were there any in each subsequent six-month interval until 18 months prior to death or medical retirement. Starting at 18 months, however, the AIDS patients spent four fewer days plucking, which amounted to 10 percent fewer kilograms of tea plucked; at the time of termination, they exhibited nearly an eight-day and 19 percent disadvantage in time spent plucking.

We can also get a sense of the adverse productivity effects of AIDS by looking at improvements that result from antiretroviral treatment (ART).

Since the medicine suppresses the HIV virus and slows disease progression, it should improve patients' overall health and their ability to engage in physical activity. If we see that this improved health leads to improvements in labor force participation or productivity, then we can assume that declines in health may have the opposite effect and decrease the likelihood of working and productivity on the job.

A study in Western Kenya exploits longitudinal data and a program's eligibility rule for ART that uses biomarkers not easily affected by patient behavior in the late stages of the disease to estimate the impact of treatment on employment outcomes (Thirumurthy, Zivin, and Goldstein 2008). It found that within six months of treatment initiation, the likelihood of working increased by 20 percent and weekly hours worked by 35 percent.

In India, another study followed patients before and after they received treatment, all of whom were initiating treatment at different times, given the course of their disease (Thirumurthy and others 2011). It also found increases in labor force participation, hours worked, and income six months after treatment, effects that persisted even 24 months after treatment.

Risky sex can also indirectly affect future productivity by increasing the risk of pregnancy. National surveys of adolescents in Burkina Faso, Ghana, Malawi, and Uganda found that premarital sex while in school is associated with an increase of two to three times in girls' odds of dropping out before completing secondary school, relative to a situation without premarital sex, even after controlling for a number of characteristics such as ethnicity, religion, household wealth, and late school entry (Biddlecom and others 2008).

Alcohol

Unlike the other risky behaviors discussed, the intoxication effects of illicit drugs and alcohol impair judgment right away and can carry an immediate risk of morbidity and mortality. Worldwide, nearly 4 percent of deaths have been attributed to alcohol (Rehm and others 2009). Nearly one in every five deaths due to poisoning have been attributed to alcohol, as were approximately 11 percent and 16 percent of all deaths due to self-inflicted injuries and drowning (WHO 2011).

These risks are also apparent in studies that have focused on a particular context. In India, for example, over 20 percent of all traumatic brain injuries and 60 percent of all injuries in emergency rooms can be traced to excessive alcohol consumption (Benegal and others 2002; Gururaj 2002, cited in Benegal 2005). In the United States, there is a sharp, discrete increase in mortality at the age of 21, the minimum drinking age mandated by law, when the number of deaths with an explicit mention of alcohol increases by 35 percent. At this age, deaths due to motor vehicle accidents suddenly increase by 15 percent, while the suicide rate jumps by 16 percent (Carpenter and Dobkin 2009).

Disease burden of alcohol

While moderate consumption of alcohol can increase the amount of good cholesterol in the body, excessive consumption raises levels of triglycerides, which increases the likelihood of heart disease. Alcohol damages cells in the liver, leading to a host of liver diseases, such as fatty liver disease, alcoholic hepatitis, and cirrhosis. According to the American Cancer Society, scientists do not completely understand the way alcohol causes cancer. It could raise the levels of certain hormones, or it could become carcinogenic because of the way the body metabolizes it.

Worldwide, alcohol seems to play a large mediating role in deaths due to these diseases (table 3.3). Alcohol, for example, has been implicated in approximately one-third of all epilepsy-related deaths (WHO 2011). Although moderate alcohol consumption can have protective effects for cerebrovascular disease, ischemic heart disease, and diabetes, the net effect tends to be harmful. While table 3.3 does not disaggregate the population attributable fractions by gender, women do appear to enjoy the protective effects of alcohol, most likely because they are less likely to engage in excessive consumption.

Table 3.3 Alcohol-Attributable Deaths

	Deaths attributed to alcohol (population attributable fractions)
Cirrhosis	48.3
Esophageal cancer	30.9
Liver cancer	30.3
Mouth and oropharynx cancers	23.0
Hypertensive heart disease	13.3
Breast cancer	7.4
Other neoplasms	7.0
Colon and rectum cancers	2.7
Cerebrovascular disease	1.9
Ischemic heart disease	1.2
Unipolar depressive disorder	1.5
Diabetes mellitus	−0.1

Source: Data are from the World Health Organization (WHO) 2011.

Links to other health-related risk-taking

A recent meta-analysis of 40 studies—most of which were conducted in the United States—found that alcohol drinkers were only 50–60 percent as likely to adhere to their HIV treatment; problem drinkers were even less likely to be adherent (Hendershot and others 2009). Some evidence links alcohol and risky sex, although a causal relationship has not been established; both excessive alcohol consumption and risky sex may stem from an underlying preference to take certain types of risk. A multisite study survey of intravenous drug users in 11 middle- and low-income countries and cities[6] estimated that men and women who had engaged in hazardous drinking (more than 14 drinks per week for men and seven per week for women) were twice as likely to report multiple sexual partners, and 1.5 times as likely to report not using a condom with their primary sexual partner, even after adjusting for gender, age, type of injected drug used, and self-reported HIV status (Arasteh and Des Jarlais 2010).

Negative impact on subsequent human capital accumulation

In the United States, a longitudinal study found that individuals who reported frequent drinking (two or more occasions in the week prior to the survey) or frequent drunkenness (six or more drinks on four or more occasions) while in high school ended up finishing 2.3 fewer years of college (Cook and Moore 1993). Since the time devoted to drinking and the time spent studying might be decided jointly (and thus might not reflect a causal relationship), the authors of the study only examined the variation in drinking that could be explained by the beer tax and the minimum purchase age in an individual's state, which could arguably be unrelated to decisions related to studying other than through their impact on drinking.

Since alcohol can affect human capital investment in the long run, we might also expect that it would lower contemporaneous productivity. A review of the literature for the United States cites small-scale experiments mentioned by Irving Fisher, an American economist in the early 20th century, in which four typesetters were divided into two groups for a four-day period (Cook and Moore 2000). One group was given drinks, while the other two typesetters served as the control group; the study concluded that drinking three glasses of beer per day reduced productivity by 10 percent.

There is not much empirical evidence outside of this small experiment, however, for a causal link between alcohol abuse and productivity. Another study that relied on nationally representative cross-sectional data and variation in beer taxes in the United States to generate variation in drinking did not find significant impacts of alcohol on the likelihood that a person was employed or unemployed, even though simple comparisons between those with a drinking problem and those who abstain from drinking do show that drinkers are less likely to be employed (Mullahy and Sindelar 1996). However, these comparisons do not take into account the possibility that people who cannot obtain or maintain employment decide to drink.

Illicit Drugs

Although illicit drugs should also have disastrous consequences for users' health, it is more difficult to empirically estimate their health consequences. Prevalence data on drug use are scant, as are surveys among a representative population in which people freely admit to illicit drug use. This makes it difficult to estimate the relative risks of dying or contracting disease from drug use. Typically, we must rely on special surveys in places like prisons, drug-treatment centers, or medical settings, which target drug users, to estimate the prevalence of drug-related deaths.

From country reports that only count deaths from overdose and trauma, the United Nations Office on Drugs and Crime (UNODC) estimates that there were from 99,000 to 253,000 deaths from illicit drug use in 2010 (UNODC 2012), and substantial regional variation was observed. Drug use accounted for 1 in 20 deaths in North America and Oceania, 1 in a 100 deaths in Asia, 1 in 110 deaths in Europe, 1 in 150 deaths in Africa, and 1 in 200 deaths in South America. While these mortality figures translate into 0.4 percent of global deaths, they are small in comparison to what has been attributed to alcohol (3.8 percent) and tobacco (8.7 percent) (Degenhardt and Hall 2012).

These data, however, should be interpreted with caution. First, while the data for North America and Europe are representative, the data from Asia cover only 8 percent of the population, and the data from the Africa region cover only 1 percent. Second, there is rarely any standardization across surveys in what constitutes a drug user (for example, someone who has injected drugs at some point in the past, someone who has injected drugs in the past 12 months) or in representativeness of the samples. Moreover, countries with higher measured prevalence may be countries with better monitoring and reporting systems, not necessarily countries with worse drug problems.

Nevertheless, from these limited data, we can infer that drug use leads to serious illnesses. Table 3.4 presents drug use prevalence, HIV prevalence, and hepatitis C among drug users for selected countries from systematic reviews of studies that examined injecting drug use, HIV, and hepatitis C (Mathers and others 2008; Nelson and others 2011). Little relationship is evident between estimated drug prevalence and HIV prevalence among users. Indonesia, for example, reports a drug use prevalence of 0.14 percent,

Table 3.4 Drug Use and Disease Prevalence, Selected Countries

Country	Prevalence of injecting drug use (percent)	Prevalence of HIV among people who inject drugs (percent)	Prevalence of hepatitis C among people who inject drugs (percent)
Azerbaijan	5.21	13.00	n.a.
Georgia	4.19	1.63	58.20
Russian Federation	1.78	37.15	72.50
Malaysia	1.33	10.30	67.10
Canada	1.30	13.40	64.00
United States	0.96	15.57	73.40
Kazakhstan	0.96	9.20	58.80
Brazil	0.67	48.00	63.90
Switzerland	0.65	1.40	78.30
Tajikistan	0.45	14.70	61.30
Finland	0.45	0.20	21.10
United Kingdom	0.39	2.30	50.50
Thailand	0.38	42.50	89.80
Spain	0.31	39.70	79.60
Argentina	0.29	49.70	54.60
Vietnam	0.25	33.85	74.10
China	0.25	12.30	67.00
Burma	0.23	42.60	79.20
Germany	0.17	2.90	75.00
Nepal	0.15	41.39	87.30
Pakistan	0.14	10.80	84.00
Indonesia	0.14	42.50	77.30
Moldova	0.14	17.00	42.70
Armenia	0.10	13.40	n.a.
Bangladesh	0.03	1.35	48.20
India	0.02	11.15	41.00
Cambodia	0.02	22.80	n.a.

Sources: Data are from Mathers and others (2008) for drug use prevalence and HIV prevalence; Nelson and others (2011) for hepatitis C prevalence.

Note: n.a. = not applicable.

but among this population, an estimated HIV prevalence of more than 42 percent. However, 0.65 percent of the population of Switzerland injects drugs, while only 1.4 percent has HIV. Perhaps wealthier countries can afford both more drugs and more disposable needles. The third column, however, reports prevalence of hepatitis C (which can lead to cirrhosis or cancer of the liver), and here we see a substantial proportion of users infected in all countries (Nelson and others 2011). Sometimes, the medium of infection is an infected needle or syringe. Some drugs such as cocaine or methamphetamines can also stimulate users or reduce their inhibitions, which can lead to more risk-taking, such as unprotected sex with multiple partners.

Summary

In all of these cases, we find that engaging in a risky behavior carries considerable risk for both dying early and living many years with compromised health. The consequent diseases are expensive to treat, even in low-income, resource-poor settings, and they exert a significant toll on individuals' productivity. In most low-income countries, it is difficult to formally insure against these costly consequences, given the rarity of both health insurance and public or private disability benefits. According to the World Development Indicators, 75 percent of private expenditure on health was financed through out-of-pocket payments in low-income countries in 2011. Accordingly, individuals take on substantial financial burdens when health consequences materialize.

Consequences to Immediate Peers

These health and financial consequences are not limited to the individuals engaging in risky behaviors. These behaviors also generate substantial spillovers to family members or coworkers. Sometimes, the spillovers result from physical proximity, as in secondhand smoke, road accidents, or the transmission of health in the womb. Sometimes, the impact of these behaviors on others is more indirect, for example, through their negative impact on household income or expenditures. In either case, these peers who suffer the consequences of someone else's behavior are typically not compensated for the troubles that befall them, which is the very definition of an externality. The following sections quantify these externalities for each behavior.

Smoking

One of the most obvious externalities generated by smoking is secondhand smoke, which leads to considerable rates of mortality and morbidity to both family members and coworkers. In a global study employing population attributable fractions to estimate secondhand smoke's contribution to disease burdens, 40 percent of children, 33 percent of male nonsmokers, and 35 percent of female nonsmokers were exposed in 2004 (Öberg and others 2011); 603,000 deaths could be attributed to secondhand smoke. Women accounted for 47 percent of deaths, with the rest of these deaths spread across children (28 percent) and men (26 percent). The morbidity toll, however, fell the hardest on children, who accounted for 61 percent of all disability-adjusted life years lost, with close to 6 million children in 2004 suffering from lower respiratory infections induced by secondhand smoke.

Secondhand smoking and children

Figure 3.2 presents the fraction of youth ages 13 to 15 exposed to secondhand smoke in the home for selected countries (see Eriksen, Mackay, and Ross 2012 for a complete listing). In most of the 120 countries included in the Global Youth Tobacco Survey, at least 20 percent of youth inhale secondhand smoke in the home.

Figure 3.2   Fraction of Youth Exposed to Secondhand Smoke in the Home, Selected Countries

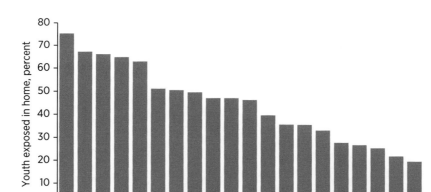

Source: Exposure data from Eriksen, Mackay, and Ross, World Tables 2012.

Note: The figure summarizes data from the Global Youth Tobacco Survey question, "During the past seven days, on how many days has anyone smoked inside your home, in your presence?"

Some suggestive evidence indicates that this secondhand smoke, in addition to causing tobacco-related illnesses in children, also depresses their cognitive performance. A longitudinal study using pregnancies occurring between 1960 and 1967 in California found a significant association between parental smoking and scores on two of four cognitive skills tests, which persisted even after the inclusion of controls for parental income, education, and prenatal smoking (Bauman, Flewelling, and LaPrelle 1991). The mechanism behind this relationship, however, remains unclear. We do not know, for example, whether secondhand smoke deprives children's brains of oxygen, whether it is associated illnesses such as respiratory infections that impair cognitive performance, or whether parents who smoke tend to be less effective in fostering the cognitive development of their children.

We do know that parental smoking—at least the smoking of mothers—does have a biological impact on children while they are still in the womb. The evidence comes from both randomized control trials and the natural experiments that often result from changes in the price of cigarettes. In one trial in the United States, pregnant smokers were randomized into a group that received standard prenatal care or another group that also received counseling to quit smoking during their pregnancies. To estimate the impact of maternal smoking on birth outcomes from this experiment, we can look at the ratio of the direct impact of the counseling on birth outcomes to the impact of the counseling on maternal smoking (the Wald estimator in econometrics). A study that analyzed this experiment's data in this way found a smoking effect of 400 grams in birth weight, or nearly 0.9 of a pound (Permutt and Hebel 1989). Given the evidence on the detrimental impact of low birth weight on outcomes later in life, such as educational attainment and wages (Black, Devereux, and Salvanes 2007; Oreopoulos and others 2008; Royer 2009), this health discrepancy that emerges among children of smokers and nonsmokers very early in life could translate into permanent differences in terms of adult health and income.

Outside of the deliberate manipulation of experiments, we need to rely on forces that influence whether pregnant women smoke but that do not affect birth outcomes directly. Changes in cigarette prices can often do this, since they tend to follow a change in an excise tax specific to cigarettes. In another study, researchers used the census of all births in the United States, which records the smoking status of the mother, and examined what happened to maternal smoking and birth outcomes after a change in states' excise taxes on cigarettes (Evans and Ringel 1999). They found a similar impact on birth weight, namely, a detrimental smoking effect of 353 to 594 grams.

Secondhand smoke and coworkers

Since smokers generally do not limit their habit to the home, smoking could also affect their coworkers if nothing prevents exposure to secondhand smoke, such as a smoking room or a ban on smoking in the workplace. The Taiwanese study discussed earlier that examined impacts within the workplace (Tsai and others 2005) also tried to monetize the burden on nonsmoking coworkers. Earlier studies among the police force in Hong Kong, China, had established a relationship for nonsmokers between respiratory problems and the number of coworkers who smoked (Lam and others 2000), and between this kind of passive smoking and sick leave (McGhee and others 2000). Taking these parameters and applying them to the workforce in Taiwan, China, the authors of the Taiwanese study calculated the value of sick leave induced by secondhand smoke to be US$81 million per year, nearly 44 percent of the direct impact of smoking on sick leave for smokers.

This exposure to secondhand smoke by other family members and coworkers translates into substantial health care costs and days away from work. The police force study from Hong Kong, China, for example, combined population attributable fractions and secondhand smoke exposures calculated from local data with information on the costs of treating smoking-related illnesses in hospitals. The results suggest that the health care expenditures and the value of missed work days totaled approximately US$156 million in 1998 (McGhee and others 2000).

These externalities are not limited to direct impacts on health. The additional spending on buying cigarettes and treating smoking-related diseases also translates into less money to spend on food, education, and other essentials for the household members, particularly children, who do not smoke.

Obesity

Obesity has a direct, biological effect on children. A study in Sweden used all pregnancy records in the Swedish Medical Birth Registry from 1992 to 2001 (over 800,000 births). The registry also contains information on maternal height and weight in early pregnancy and thus permits a prospective examination of the impact of maternal obesity on later pregnancy events and birth outcomes (Cedergren 2004). The risk of delivering a baby who is large for gestational age (2 standard deviations above the mean weight), for example, was 2.2 times higher for obese women compared to women whose body mass index fell in the normal range, even after controlling for maternal age, education, smoking behavior, and parity. There seems to be a dose response: the risk of delivering a baby who is large for gestational age for morbidly obese women was close to 3.8 times higher.

Data availability limits our ability to design a similar prospective study in low-income countries, but we can take advantage of retrospective data that span multiple countries to check for associations between maternal obesity and infant health. A recent study, for example, pooled data from the most recent Demographic and Health Surveys in 27 Sub-Saharan African countries, which ask about births in the previous five years and which measure the current heights and weights of people living in sample households. After excluding women who had become pregnant again and women who were within three months postpartum, and controlling for potential confounders such as maternal age, wealth, education, area of residence, and parity, the authors found a strong association between obesity and infant mortality. Babies born to overweight mothers had a 22 percent higher chance of dying, while babies born to obese mothers displayed a 46 percent higher risk (Creswell and others 2012). Ideally, mothers' weights would have been measured before they became pregnant to rule out an alternative hypothesis that involves reverse causation (for example, women gain weight in response to the death of their child) or the influence of some third factor that influenced both weight gain during or after pregnancy and the risk of infant death (for example, gestational diabetes). To address this, the authors show that the downward trends in body mass index associated with the time elapsed since birth were identical for both mothers who lost their children and mothers whose infants survived.

Even after birth, parental obesity increases the likelihood that a child will grow into an obese adult, although it is not possible to disentangle intergenerational transmission of lifestyle from genetic inheritability of obesity. A study used data from the United States to calculate the risks of childhood obesity related to parental obesity. Children, at all ages from 1 to 17, were 2.8 to 3.6 times as likely to be obese if their mother was obese and 2.4 to 2.9 times as likely to be obese if their father was obese (Whitaker and others 1997), with the odds increasing if both parents were obese.

Risky Sex

Given some of the mechanisms through which diseases like HIV/AIDS spread (for example, unprotected sex and exchange of bodily fluids), risky sex poses a threat for disease transmission to individuals' sexual partners and to babies of infected mothers during pregnancy, labor, delivery, or breastfeeding. In the absence of any medical interventions, for example, mother-to-child transmission rates range from 15 to 45 percent (WHO 2013).

The increased mortality and declines in productivity that accompany HIV/AIDS can also have a large impact on how other household members spend their time. Again, we can examine this impact by looking at what happens when AIDS patients receive treatment. In the Kenyan ART studies, when adult AIDS patients were given treatment for more than 100 days, young boys ages 8 to 12 years benefited enormously when their parent(s) could get back to work. The boys were 21.4 percentage points (or 30 percent) less likely to work, and they worked 8.5 (or 70 percent) fewer hours per week (Thirumurthy and others 2008).

The same study also examined how different family members allocated their time within the household (d'Adda and others 2009). It finds that this treatment increased the time female patients spent on physically demanding chores, such as fetching water, which increased by two hours per week (or 64 percent), and collecting firewood, which increased by one hour (or 46 percent). This increase, in turn, reduced the burden on children in the household. Boys in the household devoted 2.4 (81 percent) fewer hours to housework, while girls spent 0.86 (37 percent) fewer hours fetching water. This allowed children to increase their school attendance by six hours per week, nearly an entire day of school (Zivin, Thirumurthy, and Goldstein 2009).

These impacts of treatment suggest that illness had a detrimental impact on children within the household who had to assume the burden of housework that their sick parents or relatives could not perform and who had to forgo going to school. Once parents succumb to the disease, the children they leave behind as orphans suffer even more. According to estimates from the Joint United Nations Programme on HIV/AIDS and the World Health Organization (WHO), in 2009, more than 16 million children in Sub-Saharan Africa had been orphaned by HIV/AIDS (UNAIDS 2010). A longitudinal survey in KwaZulu-Natal, South Africa, had followed nearly 11,000 households since 2000 and can help illuminate what happens to children following the death of a parent. Although when fathers died between survey rounds, their children completed less schooling and parents spent less on their school-related expenditures, this effect disappears once the household's socioeconomic status is taken into account (Case and Ardington 2006). However, children who lost their mother completed a quarter of a year less schooling and experienced a 15 to 20 percent decline in their education-related expenses, relative to children who did not lose their mother. One empirical pattern that supports a causal interpretation of this association between maternal death and schooling investment is the lack of a relationship in the longitudinal data between schooling attainment and future maternal deaths. Thus, there does not seem to be something that makes these households different prior to the maternal death, such as a lower emphasis placed on the education of children.

A study from another surveillance site in South Africa estimates that the costs of funerals amount to 40 percent of average annual total household expenditure when an adult dies (Case and Menendez 2009). This increase in spending immediately following death triggers a number of other pathologies in subsequent periods, such as 20 percent lower expenditure per person, more symptoms of depression and anxiety among adults, and lower school enrollment among children. These results persist even when taking into account whether the deceased's income was financially important for the household. These adverse impacts exhibit a dose response as they increase with the amount spent on funerals.

Alcohol and Illicit Drugs

The impaired judgment that results from alcohol and illicit drugs can have immediate consequences for violence and crime. They can also generate lifelong consequences for children.

Alcohol and violence

Worldwide, alcohol has been implicated in more than 30 percent of all deaths due to violence and 21 percent of all fatal road traffic accidents (WHO 2011), and these impacts appear more severe in low-income settings. Figure 3.3 plots the fraction of all deaths from violence that have been attributed to alcohol in 2004; among the countries for which the WHO reports data, the poorer countries are more likely to fall in the set with higher values. In Guatemala, for example, alcohol had been implicated in nearly 44 percent of deaths due to violence.

A study in Australia estimates that among all hospitalizations due to interpersonal violence and road accidents, approximately 21 percent could be attributed to alcohol (Laslett and others 2010). In police data from two states (Western Australia and New South Wales), alcohol had been implicated in 42 to 44 percent of all assaults in 2004. The costs to victims in these cases include the opportunity cost of calling the police, fees for the emergency room and any subsequent medical costs, damage to personal belongings, lost output, and counseling; these add up to an average cost to victims after 12 months of US$1,615. According to the same police records, alcohol was involved in 42 to 50 percent of all domestic violence incidents.

Another study in the United States also documents a causal link between alcohol consumption and crime. It exploits the minimum drinking age law and data on arrests in California and finds a discrete jump in arrest rates for nuisance and violent crimes when individuals reach the minimum drinking age (Carpenter and Dobkin 2013).

Other studies also suggest a relationship between alcohol consumption and domestic violence. Using cross-sectional data from Uganda's Demographic and Health Survey, one study estimates that relative to women who report that their partners do not drink, women reporting occasional or frequent drunkenness of their partners were approximately 2.5 and 6 times as likely to report an act of intimate physical partner violence, such as being punched with a fist or choked deliberately (Tumwesigye and others 2012). Another study in three villages in

Figure 3.3 Alcohol-Attributable Deaths Due to Violence

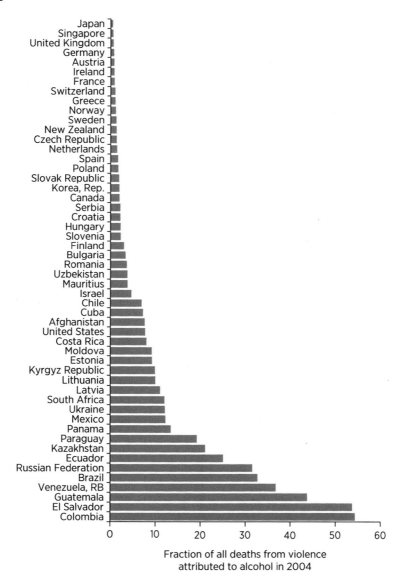

Fraction of all deaths from violence
attributed to alcohol in 2004

Source: Data are from WHO 2011.

southern India found a relationship between drunkenness and wife-beating in focus group discussions, in addition to a statistically significant association between the proportion of household expenditures devoted to alcohol and wife-beating in household survey data (Rao 1997). Similarly, the WorldSAFE study examined the association between regular drinking and the likelihood that a woman has ever experienced physical violence by her partner in three urban areas in India and one urban area in Chile. It found that after adjusting for basic demographics, mental health, and employment disparities between spouses, women with partners who drink regularly were 2.5 to 7 times as likely to experience violence relative to women whose partners never drank (Jeyaseelan and others 2004).

While it is possible that none of these relationships is causal—whatever unobserved trait could be driving the alcohol consumption could also be responsible for the domestic violence—some evidence suggests that some abuse is indeed induced by alcohol. Another U.S. study, using data from the National Family Violence Surveys in 1976 and 1985, takes advantage of the variation in drinking that can be explained by beer taxes. It finds that females are fairly responsive; a 1 percent increase in the beer tax led to a 0.33 percent decrease in the likelihood that they commit severe violence toward a child in 1976,[7] with a reduced—but still statistically significant—effect in the 1985 round as well (Markowitz and Grossman 2000). As with the other studies that have tried to isolate a causal effect of alcohol by using variation in taxes, we still might worry that areas with higher beer taxes are precisely the areas where people care more about public safety or the safety of children and that these people may be less prone to abusing their children.

Lifelong consequences for children
One established causal effect of alcohol is fetal alcohol syndrome, when mothers drink to excess during pregnancy. This is one of the leading causes of mental retardation, marked by severe learning disabilities, abnormal facial features, and growth problems. While not all children exposed to alcohol in utero will develop this syndrome, the results from a natural experiment in Sweden suggest that alcohol exposure in utero can have long-term effects that extend beyond childhood (Nilsson 2008).

Sweden briefly experimented in several counties with selling strong beer through grocery stores in the late 1960s, which sharply increased alcohol consumption, especially among youth who were legally barred from purchasing the beverage in other outlets before the age of 21; the policy was subsequently reversed because of the magnitude of this increase. To estimate the impact of this policy experiment on later life outcomes, we can compare people who were in utero during the experiment and whose mothers were below the age of 21 to children in nonparticipating counties and to older or younger children in the same counties who were not in utero during the policy experiment. These comparisons suggest that the increased alcohol exposure induced by the policy experiment decreased high school graduation rates by 4 percentage points and graduation rates from higher education by 2.5 percentage points. Thus, it should not be surprising that the exposed cohorts also earned 24 percent less on average, were 7 percentage points more likely to have no income earnings at all, and relied on welfare 3.6 percentage points more often.

While it makes sense that drug use during pregnancy could also have adverse effects for children, it is difficult to find studies that adequately control for other possible confounding factors (for example, an expecting mother who takes cocaine may also neglect to go for prenatal care), and meta-analyses of the association between birth outcomes and cannabis use, and birth outcomes and cocaine use, note the associations but caution about causal interpretations (English and others 1997; Hulse and others 1997).

Summary

Each of these risky behaviors can directly influence the health of family workers and coworkers through secondhand smoke, their adverse impacts on babies in utero that can persist throughout their lifetime, disease transmission to sexual partners, or violence and other additional risk-taking triggered by these behaviors, such as drunk driving. The consequences extend beyond the individuals. Their immediate peers also experience declines in productivity. Children suffer a decline in the amount invested in their human capital, either because they must forgo schooling due to a sick parent who cannot work, or because exposure in utero has put them on a lower trajectory in terms of cognitive abilities. Given that these injured parties are not and typically cannot be compensated for their losses (for example, coworkers of smokers are not offered more health care services, nor are there remedial education programs targeting children whose mothers drank during pregnancy), policy makers interested in maximizing social welfare need to develop and implement policies and programs that can decrease the frequency of these risky behaviors or force individuals who continue to engage in them to internalize the externalities that they generate (see chapters 4 and 5 for a review of interventions that try to do this).

Societal Consequences

Even when medical treatment requires considerable out-of-pocket payments, these risky behaviors can trigger consequences that go beyond the household and immediate peers.

- First, health systems will still bear some of the costs of treatment, especially since some of the health consequences can be catastrophic, and in the absence of an established system of health insurance, will be beyond the financial means of most households in middle- and low-income countries. These are typically classified as the *direct costs* of risky behaviors.
- Second, the excess mortality and morbidity associated with these behaviors lead to premature deaths, early exits from the labor force, and decreased productivity while working, all of which can reduce aggregate productivity and economic growth. These impacts are typically classified as *indirect costs*.

While individuals bear some of these costs through reductions in their private earnings, they can have a broader impact to the extent that they contribute to a shrinking of a country's total economic output, which means fewer products and services in an economy, in addition to less tax revenue.

It is important to note, however, that none of the studies have put a cost on the human capital losses suffered by the children who are directly affected when the adults in their family engage in risky behavior. Smoking, for instance, not only depresses current economic output through its adverse productivity on smokers and their coworkers; it also decreases future output by compromising babies' health in utero, which in turn has an adverse impact on their lifetime education and employment trajectories. Similarly, HIV/AIDS can be debilitating for those who have the disease; at the same time, it can wreck the future prospects for their children. Thus, we should consider the societal costs discussed as lower bounds of the true societal costs generated when individuals engage in behaviors that put their health at risk.

Smoking

Because tobacco-related illnesses typically require hospitalization, the direct costs of smoking can be high. Although smokers can benefit from fewer medical interventions in poor countries, the financial implications of treatment can still exert a toll on health systems.

Direct costs
Figure 3.4 presents the total direct costs of smoking from a number of middle- and low-income countries in 2010. These costs, which combine public and private spending, can be considered the total opportunity costs of treating smoking-related illnesses. To put some of these figures in perspective, the US$5.7 billion spent in Mexico, for example, accounted for over 10 percent of all health care expenditures between 2003 and 2008 (Ericksen, Mackay, and Ross 2012). The US$114 billion spent by Chile in 2008 could

Figure 3.4 Direct Costs of Smoking

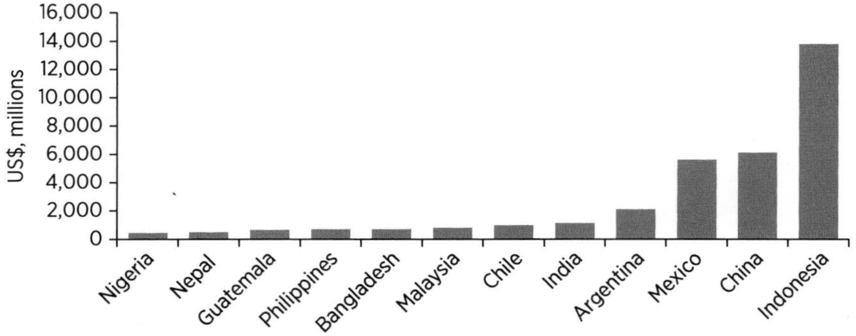

Source: Data are from Ericksen, Mackay, and Ross 2012.

have paid for its entire public safety program, and Malaysia's direct costs of US$922 million could have funded its entire rural development program.

Indirect costs of smoking

The direct costs of smoking, however, are typically dwarfed by the indirect costs of lost productivity. In Bangladesh, for example, the indirect costs of tobacco-related illnesses were more than double the direct costs (figure 3.5) and nearly double any benefit that could arise from tax revenue or wages in the tobacco sector. The net costs to society in 2003 were US$44 million (WHO 2005).

A similar pattern was observed in data from China's National Health Services Survey. While the direct costs totaled US$6.2 billion, the indirect costs—which included the costs of transportation and caregivers used when dealing with smoking-related illnesses—reached nearly US$22.7 billion (Yang and others 2011). We might even expect these figures to be underestimates of the indirect costs attributable to smoking, since the analysis omitted the impacts of secondhand smoke and used the total number of days a person was hospitalized to proxy for the number of days missed from work.

A study in India, however, yielded higher direct costs, most likely because data were not available to calculate the value of premature deaths (John, Sung, and Max 2009). In 2004, the smoking attributable fractions for the male population older than 35 years in India were quite high for respiratory diseases (30.04 percent), tuberculosis (33.43), cardiovascular diseases (17.65), and cancers (38.47). These translated into costs that exceeded the total excise tax revenue collected on tobacco products in the same year. Direct health expenditures totaled US$834 million. Expenditures on transportation and caregivers for each inpatient

Figure 3.5 Direct and Indirect Costs of Smoking in Bangladesh

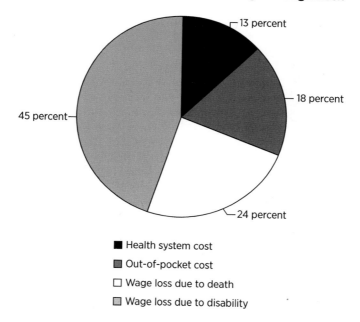

13 percent

18 percent

45 percent

24 percent

■ Health system cost
▨ Out-of-pocket cost
☐ Wage loss due to death
▥ Wage loss due to disability

Source: Data are from WHO 2005.

or outpatient health care visit amounted to another US$65 million, while income lost due to work absences when hospitalized or seeking outpatient care totaled US$314 million. Again, since we expect individuals with these conditions to miss work even when they are not seeking medical attention, this should be considered a lower bound for the value of lost productivity.

The study in Taiwan, China, that estimated days of lost work from sick leave and smoking breaks found that when priced at average wage per hour, these lost work days added up to US$917 million per year (Tsai and others 2005). Since these workers were presumably not fined for taking smoking breaks or penalized with lower salaries, this can simply be thought of as a pure loss in output.

Obesity

Because they entail frequent use of primary care services, high medical expenditures, and productivity losses during prime working ages, the chronic diseases that accompany obesity could both burden health systems in low-income countries and depress aggregate productivity.

Direct Costs of Obesity

A study focused on Latin America, for example, used estimates from Costa Rica of an association between diabetes and excess medical visits and hospitalizations, and applied them to the total number of people afflicted with diabetes and the number of medical visits and hospitalizations per inhabitant in Latin America. It found that in 2000, diabetes accounted for about one-third of all consultations and one-third of all days spent in the hospital (Barceló and others 2003).

In China, where state expenditures account for a large majority of health care costs, the costs associated with hospitalizations, outpatient services, and prescription drugs for cancer, coronary heart disease, stroke, hypertension, and diabetes accounted for nearly US$11.74 billion, when relative risks from U.S. studies and prevalence data from China were combined to estimate the fraction of these diseases attributable to diet (Popkin and others 2001). This finding corresponds to more than 22 percent of health care costs in 1995 or 1.6 percent of GDP. In India, where most health care expenditures are financed out of pocket, the direct costs associated with these diseases stood at US$1.10 billion, which was nearly 14 percent of all expenditure on hospitalization, outpatient services, and drugs, or 0.35 percent of GDP.

In the United States, the direct costs of treating obesity-related conditions ranged from US$92 to $117 billion in 2002. The indirect costs from missed work and future earnings losses due to premature death were $56 billion per year (Haskins, Paxson, and Donahue 2006). To the extent that some obese people do not seek adequate medical attention (for example, if they are more likely to be poor), these are likely to be underestimates of the total costs required to deal with the health consequences of obesity. Indeed, a study that tried to isolate the causal impact of obesity on medical spending (as opposed to just the correlation) using only the variation in weight that can be explained by genetics (rather than poverty, for example) found that medical care costs of adult obesity in 2005 were US$190.2 billion, or 20.6 percent of all health expenditures in the United States (Cawley and Meyerhoefer 2012).

Indirect costs of obesity

In low-income countries, however, the indirect costs of productivity losses are much higher relative to the aggregate costs of treatment, perhaps because the costs of sustained treatment are so high in wealthier countries. Another China study, for example, examined costs incurred by health care facilities (which were either reimbursed by the state or from private fees from patients or insurance plans) for five diseases linked to obesity: cancer, coronary heart disease, stroke, hypertension, and diabetes (Popkin and others 2006). The study used relative risks calculated from U.S. studies to estimate the fraction of these disease burdens attributable to obesity and its impact on sick leave in China. The findings indicate that in 2000, the total costs from the prevalence of overweight and obesity among Chinese adults amounted to over 4 percent of gross national product, with indirect costs—specifically, sick leave—accounting for the lion's share of these costs (figure 3.6).

Similarly, in India, the annual productivity costs in 1995 associated with premature deaths alone—US$2.25 billion—were more than twice as high as the annual costs to the health care system (Popkin and others 2001).

Comparing the costs attributable to cardiovascular disease and diabetes in North and South America provides more direct evidence of this difference in the relative costs of treatment and productivity losses across high- and low-income countries. In a group of countries that includes Canada, Cuba, and the United States, productivity losses added up to only 65 percent of the direct costs of cardiovascular disease (Bonilla-Chacín 2012). In the group that contained all other countries in the region, however, productivity costs were almost twice as large as direct costs. Similarly, in North America, the indirect costs associated with diabetes accounted for 36 percent of total costs, whereas in Central and South America, they amounted to 68 and 85 percent, respectively, of all costs.

All of these estimates from low-income countries, however, rely on existing data on the prevalence of these diseases. Since a person must make contact with the formal health care system and be diagnosed appropriately in order to contribute to these estimates of prevalence, and since the use of informal health providers (Banerjee, Deaton, and Duflo 2004;

Figure 3.6 Direct and Indirect Costs of Overweight and Obesity in China in 2000

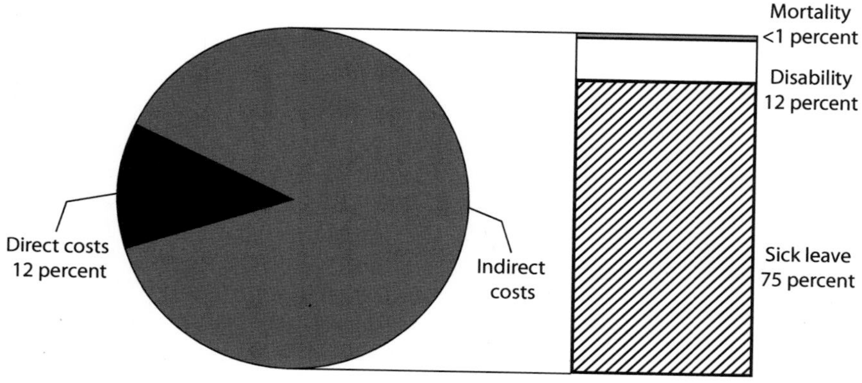

Source: Data are from Popkin and others 2006, table 9.

World Bank–IFC 2011) and poor diagnostic ability among these providers characterize many health systems in low-income countries (Das and others 2012), these prevalence estimates likely underestimate the burden of disease. Indeed, the International Diabetes Foundation estimates fairly high numbers of undiagnosed cases in many of these countries. Table 3.5, for example, suggests that the number of cases could increase by 29 to 83 percent (average 58 percent), depending on the country.

Table 3.5 Undiagnosed Diabetes Cases in 2012

	Diabetes prevalence	Increase in cases if undiagnosed cases were diagnosed (percent)
Afghanistan	7.6	50
Bangladesh	7.1	50
Bolivia	6.9	46
Cameroon	6.2	80
Comoros	8.4	83
Haiti	6.7	29
India	9.0	51
Kiribati	25.5	59
Kyrgyz Republic	6.3	29
Madagascar	5.1	83
Malawi	5.6	83
Nicaragua	11.6	46
Pakistan	7.9	56
Papua New Guinea	6.5	59
São Tomé and Príncipe	5.5	80
Solomon Islands	15.3	59
Sudan	9.1	56
Tajikistan	6.3	29
Togo	5.2	83
Uzbekistan	6.4	29
Vietnam	5.8	63
Yemen, Rep.	9.2	56
Zambia	5.1	83

Source: International Diabetes Foundation.
Note: The International Diabetes Foundation reports data for Sudan and South Sudan jointly.

Risky Sex

Even if governments do not intervene to address the spillovers to other household members, the direct costs of HIV/AIDS treatment can be expensive. While the costs of ART have come down to US$150 per year, HIV treatment also includes lab tests, hospital and outpatient services, and the treatment of opportunistic infections. One study estimates that average total costs per enrolled AIDS patient in 2007 for ART was US$296 (first-line medication) to US$1,151 (second-line medication) for low-income countries with GDP per capita less than or equal to US$460 and US$835 to $2,255 for lower-middle income countries with GDP per capita greater than or equal to US$2,000 (Over 2010).

These unit costs, however, can be misleading, even if we were to multiply them by the number of people requiring treatment today, because they do not take into account the fact that each HIV infection requires treatment and possibly other social policy responses in the future for as long as the person remains alive. They also do not take into account the fact that this future liability of governments includes treatment of new infections that arise. When we do consider new infections as coming with these kinds of pension-like obligations, the fiscal costs of HIV/AIDS are staggering. In Botswana, for example, the present discounted value of these costs was estimated to be 192 percent of GDP (Lule and Haacker 2012). Even if we assume that donor support remains at current levels, the liability of the government still would amount to 156 percent of GDP. This translates into approximately twice the GDP per capita for a single HIV infection under the coverage rates of the current HIV program. In Swaziland, which has the highest prevalence in the world, this total government liability adds up to 293 percent of GDP, or 3.8 times GDP per capita for every new infection.

Effects on the health system

Important primary care services could also be affected if both financial and human resources must be diverted to address HIV/AIDS. One study that combined multiple years of the Demographic and Health Surveys from 14 countries in Sub-Saharan Africa found that the countries with the highest increases in AIDS prevalence also experienced the largest deteriorations in other health services (Case and Paxson 2009). Women were much less likely to obtain any prenatal care; conditional on getting any care, they were much less likely to get the appropriate procedures, such as urine and blood tests, weight checks, and blood pressure monitoring. They were also much less likely to deliver in a clinic or with a skilled birth attendant. Their children were also more likely to remain unvaccinated.

Impact on aggregate productivity and growth

There has been some debate on the ultimate impact of AIDS on aggregate productivity and economic growth. Alwyn Young (2005), for example, used a growth model and household surveys to simulate the impact of AIDS on economic growth. He actually predicted an increase in per capita consumption in South Africa net of the decline in orphans' human capital, which arises because AIDS lowers fertility by deterring unprotected sex and making labor more scarce, thereby increasing the value of women's time outside of the home. This lower labor-to-capital ratio, in turn, increases real wages, much like what occurred following the Black Death (the Plague) in the fifteenth century. Kalemli-Ozcan and Turan (2011), however, note that Young (2005) also used fertility data from before 1990; since he would not have been able to match these data to data on HIV prevalence rates, he assigned a value of zero to prevalence before 1990. Once they restrict the analysis to the 1990–98 period and use real HIV prevalence rates, they predict a positive impact on fertility and thus a negative impact on GDP per capita.

Another study investigates Young's (2005) labor channel more directly by examining whether variation in AIDS mortality across birth cohorts tracks variation in employment and wages in South Africa. Once individuals are matched by gender, province, birth cohort, and population group, there is a negative relationship between reductions in the size of the labor force through AIDS mortality and employment and wages of those who survive (Chicoine 2012). In particular, people from high-mortality populations (for example, blacks born after 1960) experience a decline of 3 to 6 percent in wages and a decline of 1.5 to 3.5 percentage points in employment.

Others have argued that all of these analyses are focusing on a time horizon that is too short; instead, what matters for economic growth in the long run is human capital, and AIDS is devastating for human capital (Bell and others 2006). AIDS not only kills adults in their prime (wasting any human capital they acquired from their parents, from formal education, or from on-the-job training before it could be used); it also destroys their ability to invest in their children's human capital, either because they are dead or because they have less income. Children acquiring little human capital are, in turn, less able to raise children and invest in their human capital.

If we take this longer-term perspective and consider both more micro evidence on health, productivity, and human capital accumulation of children and the costs of the fiscal liabilities associated with each current and new infection, then the societal costs of risky sex far exceed the resources of most middle- and low-income countries.

Alcohol and Illicit Drugs

The costs of alcohol to society consume a nontrivial portion of GDP, with the bulk of these costs stemming from indirect losses in productivity. Table 3.6 summarizes estimates of these costs from six high-middle- and high-income countries. In Thailand, for example, these productivity losses are devastating, accounting for nearly 95 percent of all costs attributed to alcohol (Rehm and others 2009). Some countries, like Scotland and Canada, devoted substantial law enforcement resources to dealing with alcohol, which accounted for nearly one-quarter of all costs.

While comparable data for illicit drug use are lacking, from the limited evidence that we have on its impacts, it would be reasonable to speculate that both fiscal burdens could be large if prevalence of drug use continues to grow; indeed drug use jumped from the 25th to the 19th position in leading risk factors for disease between 1990 and 2010 in the Global Burden of Disease Study. Not only would drug use contribute to the fiscal liabilities of governments through the spread of HIV, hepatitis, and other infectious diseases, but their treatment may require health infrastructure such as needle and syringe programs, opioid substitution treatment, and trained medical staff to deliver such services, which are currently unavailable in low-income countries.

Summary

In addition to spending by individuals and the peers whom they affect, society also loses when individuals engage in behaviors that put their health

Table 3.6 Societal Costs of Alcohol

	France	United States	Scotland	Canada	Republic of Korea	Thailand
Total costs as percent of GDP (PPP)	1.7	2.7	1.4	1.4	3.3	1.3
Health care as percent of total costs	16.0	12.7	8.9	22.7	6.1	4.3
Law enforcement as percent of total costs	0.3	3.4	25.0	21.1	0.0	0.2
Other direct costs as percent of total costs	33.9	11.2	8.0	7.2	21.9	0.6
Indirect costs as percent of total costs	49.9	72.7	58.0	49.0	72.0	94.8

Source: Rehm and others 2009, table 4.

Note: Other direct costs include property damage and loss, administrative costs, and social work services. PPP = purchasing power parity.

at risk. While still substantial, the opportunity costs of the medical spending required to deal with the resulting diseases are far outweighed by their productivity losses in low-income countries, even though existing studies do not even take into account the future productivity losses associated with the adverse effects that children face when the adults in their lives engage in risky behaviors.

Conclusion

The risky behaviors examined in this volume generate large costs to the individuals engaged in the behaviors, their peers, and society more generally; and in low-income countries, the productivity losses associated with these behaviors dwarf their impact on health expenditures. It may not be analytically possible to weigh the utility that individuals derive from smoking, drinking, eating, and having sex against these consequences that accrue to their peers and society in terms of death, disease, and their financial implications; nevertheless there is a clear case for intervention. High impacts on individuals and growing incidence suggest that existing markets for insurance (if they exist) will not be able to handle the medical costs or employment losses associated with these risky behaviors. The presence of large externalities to peers and the absence of policies designed to mitigate them suggest that public intervention to prevent or reduce engagement in these behaviors can improve overall welfare. Therefore, when evaluating policies designed to prevent or curtail these risky behaviors, we need not narrowly focus on comparing the costs of an intervention to the benefits; the decision not to intervene does not make much economic sense. Instead, we can evaluate the cost-effectiveness of different policies that do tackle these behaviors, which is the focus of the next two chapters.

Notes

1. Smoking affects almost every system of the body, from the eyes and skin to the digestive system; see Eriksen, Mackay, and Ross (2012) for a detailed list with references when available. This chapter focuses on the most prevalent conditions with the most evidence for an association with smoking.
2. They empirically identify this effect by first including a smooth cohort trend and then comparing these excess mortality rates by illness condition to those experienced by women, since relatively few women served in the military during these wars.
3. They were high blood pressure, diets low in fruits, high body mass index, high fasting plasma glucose, low physical activity, diets high in sodium, diets low in

seeds and nuts, high total cholesterol, diets low in whole grains, diets low in vegetables, and diets low in seafood omega-3 fatty acids.
4. Smokers both weigh less than nonsmokers and are at higher risk for cardiovascular disease.
5. These other infections can include syphilis, gonorrhea, chancroid, chlamydia, granuloma inguinale, candidiasis, hepatitis B, herpes simplex, human papilloma virus, molluscum contagiosum, crabs, scabies, and trichomoniasis.
6. Beijing, Bogota, Hanoi, Kharkiv, Lagos, Minsk, Nairobi, Rio, Rosario, Santos, and St. Petersburg.
7. Severe violence includes any one of the following actions: kicking, biting, hitting with fist, hitting or trying to hit with something else, beating up, burning, scalding, or threatening to use or using a gun or knife on child.

References

Arasteh, Kamyar, and Don C. Des Jarlais. 2010. "Hazardous Drinking and HIV Sexual Risk Behaviors Among Injection Drug Users in Developing and Transitional Countries." *AIDS and Behavior* 14 (4): 862–69.

Aubin, Henri-Jean, Amanda Farley, Deborah Lycett, Pierre Lahmek, and Paul Aveyard. 2012. "Weight Gain in Smokers after Quitting Cigarettes: Meta-Analysis." *BMJ Open*. doi: 10.1136/bmj.e4439.

Banerjee, Abhijit, Angus Deaton, and Esther Duflo. 2004. "Health, Healthcare, and Economic Development." *American Economic Review* 94 (2): 326–30.

Baquilod, M. M., M. E. Chrisostomo, G. B. Estrada, A. G. Tan, M. C. Palatino, P. L. Adversario, E. S. Prudente, J. C. Baltazar, E. L. Matibag, P. P. Ng, E. V. Vera, and A. A. Yurekli. 2008. *Tobacco and Poverty in the Philippines*. Geneva: World Health Organization.

Barceló, Alberto, Cristian Aedo, Swapnil Rajpathak, and Sylvia Robles. 2003. "The Cost of Diabetes in Latin America and the Caribbean." *Bulletin of the World Health Organization* 81 (1): 19–27.

Bauman, Karl E., Robert L. Flewelling, and John LaPrelle. 1991. "Parental Cigarette Smoking and Cognitive Performance of Children." *Health Psychology* 10 (4): 282–88.

Bedard, Kelly, and Olivier Deschênes. 2006. "The Long Term Impact of Military Service on Health: Evidence from World War II and Korean War Veterans." *American Economic Review* 96 (1): 176–94.

Bell, Clive, Shanta Devarajan, and Hans Gersbach. 2006. "The Long-Run Economic Costs of AIDS: Theory and an Application to South Africa." *World Bank Economic Review* 20 (1): 55–89.

Benegal, V., G. Gururaj, and P. Murthy. 2002. "Project Report on a WHO Multi Centre Collaborative Project On Establishing and Monitoring Alcohol's Involvement in Casualties: 2000–01." Monograph, http://www,nimhans,kar,nic,in/Deaddiction/lit/Alcohol%20and%20%20Injuries_WHO 20Collab,pdf, accessed 10 April 2005.

Benegal, Vivek. 2005. "India: Alcohol and Public Health." *Addiction* 100 (8): 1051–56.

Biddlecom, Ann, Richard Gregory, Cynthia B. Lloyd, and Barbara S. Mensch. 2008. "Associations Between Premarital Sex and Leaving School in Four Sub-Saharan African Countries." *Studies in Family Planning* 39 (4): 337–50.

Black, Sandra E., Paul J. Devereux, and Kjell G. Salvanes. 2007. "From the Cradle to the Labor Market? The Effect of Birth Weight on Adult Outcomes." *Quarterly Journal of Economics* 122 (1): 409–39.

Boily, Marie-Claude, Rebecca F. Baggaley, Lei Wang, Benoit Masse, Richard G. White, Richard J. Hayes, and Michel Alary. 2009. "Heterosexual Risk of HIV-1 Infection per Sexual Act: Systematic Review and Meta-Analysis of Observational Studies." *Lancet Infectious Disease* 9 (2): 118–29.

Bonilla-Chacín, María Eugenia. 2012. *Promoting Healthy Living in Latin America and the Caribbean: Governance of Multi-Sectoral Aactivities to Prevent Health Risk Factors.* Washington, DC: World Bank.

Carpenter, Christopher, and Carlos Dobkin. 2009. "The Effect of Alcohol Consumption on Mortality: Regression Discontinuity Evidence from the Minimum Drinking Age." *American Economic Journal: Applied Economics* 1 (1): 164–82.

———. 2013. "The Drinking Age, Alcohol Consumption, and Crime." http://web.merage.uci.edu/~kittc/Carpenter_Dobkin_Crime_website_01192011.pdf on September 9, 2013.

Case, Anne, and Cally Ardington. 2006. "The Impact of Parental Death on School Outcomes: Longitudinal Evidence from South Africa." *Demography* 43 (3): 401–20.

Case, Anne, and Alicia Menendez. 2009. "Requiescat in Pace? The Consequences of High Priced Funerals in South Africa." Working Paper 1499, National Bureau of Econopmic Research, Cambridge, MA.

Case, Anne, and Christina Paxson. 2009. "The Impact of the AIDS Pandemic on Health Services in Africa: Evidence from Demographic and Health Surveys." Working Paper 15000, National Bureau of Economic Research, Cambridge, MA.

Cawley, John. 2004. "The Impact of Obesity on Wages." *Journal of Human Resources* 39 (2): 451–74.

Cawley, John, and Chad Meyerhoefer. 2012. "The Medical Care Costs of Obesity: An Instrumental Variables Approach." *Journal of Health Economics* 31 (1): 219–30.

Cedergren, Marie I. 2004. "Maternal Morbid Obesity and the Risk of Adverse Pregnancy Outcome." *Obstetrics and Gynecology* 103 (2): 219–24.

Chicoine, Luke. 2012. "Aids Mortality and Its Effect on the Labor Market: Evidence from South Africa." *Journal of Development Economics* 98 (2): 256–69.

Cook, Philip J., and Michael J. Moore. 1993. "Drinking and Schooling." *Journal of Health Economics* 12 (4): 411–29.

———. 2000. "Alcohol." In *Handbook of Health Economics*, edited by A. J. Culyer and J.P. Newhouse, Vol. 1, 1629–73. Elsevier.

Creswell, Jenny A., Oona M. R. Campbell, Mary J. De Silva, and Véronique Filippi. 2012. "Effect of Maternal Obesity on Neonatal Death in Sub-Saharan Africa: Multivariable Analysis of 27 National Datasets." *Lancet* 380: 1325–30.

Crisp, Arthur, Philip Sedgwick, Christine Halek, Neil Joughin, and Heather Humphrey. 1999. "Why May Teenage Girls Persist in Smoking?" *Journal of Adolescence* 22: 657–72.

d'Adda, Giovanna, Markus Goldstein, Joshua Graff Zivin, Mabel Nangami, and Harsha Thirumurthy. 2009. "ARV Treatment and Time Allocation to Household Tasks: Evidence from Kenya." *African Development Review* 21: 180–208.

Das, Jishnu, Alaka Holla, Veena Das, Manoj Mohanan, Diana Tabak, and Brian Chan. 2012. "In Urban and Rural India, a Standardized Patient Study Showed Low Levels of Provider Training and Huge Quality Gaps." *Health Affairs* 31 (12): 2774–844.

Degenhardt, Louisa, and Wayne Hall. 2012. "Extent of Illicit Drug Use and Dependence, and Their Contribution to the Global Burden of Disease." *Lancet* 379 (9810): 55–70.

English, D. R., G. K. Hulse, E., Milne, C. D. J. Holman, and C. I. Bower. 1997. "Maternal Cannabis Use and Birth Weight: A Meta-Analysis." *Addiction* 92 (11): 1553–60.

Eriksen, M., J. Mackay, and H. Ross. 2012. *The Tobacco Atlas, Fourth Edition.* Atlanta, GA: American Cancer Society and World Lung Foundation.

Evans, William N., and Jeanne S. Ringel. 1999. "Can Higher Cigarette Taxes Improve Birth Outcomes?" *Journal of Public Economics* 72 (1): 135–54.

Fox, Matthew P., Sydney Rosen, William B. MacLeod, Monique Wasunna, Margaret Bii, Ginamarie Foglia, and Jonathan L. Simon. 2004. "The Impact of HIV/AIDS on Labor Productivity in Kenya." *Tropical Medicine and International Health* 9 (3): 318–24.

Gaziano, Thomas A. 2005. "Cardiovascular Disease in the Developing World and Its Cost-Effective Management." *Circulation* 112 (23): 3547–53.

———. 2007. "Reducing the Growing Burden of Cardiovascular Disease in the Developing World." *Health Affairs* 26 (1): 13–24.

Gertler, Paul, Manisha Shah, and Stefano M. Bertozzi. 2005. "Risky Business: The Market for Unprotected Commercial Sex." *Journal of Political Economy* 113 (3): 518–50.

Haacker, Markus. 2013. "The Macroeconomic Effect of HIV/AIDS." In *Elsevier Encyclopaedia of Health Economics*, edited by Tony Culyer.

Hamermesh, Daniel, and Jeff E. Biddle. 1994. "Beauty and the Labor Market." *American Economic Review* 84 (5): 1174–94.

Haskins, Ron, Christina Paxson, and Elisabeth Donohue. 2006. "Fighting Obesity in the Public Schools." *The Future of Children Policy Brief.* Princeton University, Brookings Institution.

Hendershot, Christian S., Susan A. Stoner, David W. Pantalone, and Jane M. Simoni. 2009. "Alcohol Use and Antiretroviral Adherence: Review and Meta-Analysis." *Journal of Acquired Immune Deficiency Syndromes* 5 (2): 180–202.

Hulse, G. K., D. R. English, E. Milne, C. D. J. Holman, and C. I. Bower. 1997. "Maternal Cocaine Use and Low Birth Weight Newborns: A Meta-Analysis." *Addiction* 92 (11): 1561–70.

International Diabetes Foundation. Various years. http://www.idf.org/diabetesatlas.

Jeyaseelan L., Laura S. Sadowski, Shuba Kumar, Fatma Hassan, Laurie Ramiro, and Beatriz Vizcarra. 2004. "World Studies of Abuse in the Family Environment: Risk Factors for Physical Intimate Partner Violence." *Injury Control and Safety Promotion* 11 (2): 117–24.

John, R. M., H-Y Sung, and W. Max. 2009. "Economic Costs of Tobacco Use in India, 2004." *Tobacco Control* 18: 138–43.

Kalemli-Ozcan, Sebnem, and Belgi Turan. 2011. "HIV and Fertility Revisited." *Journal of Development Economics* 96 (1): 61–65.

Laslett, A-M., P. Catalano, Y. Chikritzhs, C. Dale, C. Doran, J. Ferris, T. Jainullabudeen, M. Livingston, S. Matthews, J. Mugavin, R. Room, M. Schlotterlein, and C. Wilkinson. 2010. *The Range and Magnitude of Alcohol's Harm to Others.* Fitzroy, Victoria: AER Centre for Alcohol Policy Research, Turning Point Alcohol and Drug Centre, Eastern Health.

Lim, Stephen S., Theo Vos, Abraham D. Flaxman, Goodarz Danaei, Kenji Shibuya, Heather Adair-Rohani, Mohammad A. AlMazroa, Markus Amann, H. Ross Anderson, and Kathryn G. Andrews. 2012. "A Comparative Risk Assessment of Burden of Disease and Injury Attributable to 67 Risk Factors and Risk Factor Clusters in 21 Regions, 1990-2010: A Systematic Analysis for the Global Burden of Disease Study 2010." *Lancet* 380 (9859): 2224–60.

Luke, Nancy. 2006. "Exchange and Condom Use in Informal Sexual Relationships in Urban Kenya." *Economic Development and Cultural Change* 54 (2): 319–48.

Lule, Elizabeth, and Markus Haacker. 2012. *The Fiscal Dimensions of HIV/AIDS in Botswana, South Africa, Swaziland, and Uganda.* Washington, DC: World Bank.

Markowitz, Sara, and Michael Grossman. 2000. "The Effects of Beer Taxes on Physical Child Abuse." *Journal of Health Economics* 19 (2): 271–82.

Mathers, Bradley M., L. Degenhardt, B. Phillips, L. Wiessing, M. Hickman, S. A. Strathdee, A. Wodak, S. Panda, M. Tyndall, A. Toufik, and R. P. Mattick. 2008. "Global Epidemiology of Injecting Drug Use and HIV Among People Who Inject Drugs: A Systematic Review." *Lancet* 372 (9651): 1733–45.

McGhee, Sarah M., Peymane Adab, Anthony J. Hedley, Tai Hing Lam, Lai Ming Ho, Richard Fielding, and Chit Ming Wong. 2000. "Passive Smoking at Work: The Short-Term Cost." *Journal of Epidemiology and Community Health* 54: 673–76.

Mullahy, John, and Jody Sindelar. 1996. "Employment, Unemployment, and Problem Drinking." *Journal of Health Economics* 15 (4): 409–34.

Nagot, Nicolas, Amadou Ouangré, Abdoulaye Ouedraogo, Michel Cartoux, Pierre Huygens, Marie Christine Defer, Tarnagda Zékiba, Nicholas Meda, and Philippe Van de Perre. 2002. "Spectrum of Commercial Sex Activity in Burkina Faso: Classification Model and Risk of Exposure to HIV." *Journal of Acquired Immune Deficiency Syndromes* 29 (5): 517–21.

Nelson, Paul K., Bradley M. Mathers, Benjamin Cowie, Holly Hagan, Don Des Jarlais, Danielle Horyniak, and Louisa Degenhardt. 2011. "Global Epidemiology of Hepatitis B and Hepatitis C in People Who Inject Drugs: Results of Systematic Reviews." *Lancet* 378 (9791): 571–83.

Neuhann, H. F., C. Warter-Neuhann, I. Lyaruu, and L. Myusa. 2002. "Diabetes Care in Kilimanjaro Region: Clinical Presentation and Problems of Patients of the Diabetes Clinic at the Regional Referral Hospital: An Inventory Before Structured Intervention." *Diabetic Medicine* 19 (12): 509–13.

Ngalula, Juliana, Mark Urassa, Gabriel Mwaluko, Raphael Isingo, and J. Ties Boerma. 2002. Health Service Use and Household Expenditure During Terminal

Illness Due to AIDS in Rural Tanzania." *Tropical Medicine and International Health* 7 (10): 873–77.

Nilsson, Peter. 2008. "Does a Pint a Day Affect Your Child's Pay? The Effect of Prenatal Alcohol Exposure on Adult Outcomes." Cemmap Working Paper No. CWP22/08, Institute for Fiscal Studies, London.

Öberg, Mattias, Marrita S. Jaakkola, Alistair Woodward, Armando Peruga, and Annette Prüss-Ustün. 2011. "Worldwide Burden of Disease from Exposure to Secondhand Smoke: A Retrospective Analysis of Data from 192 Countries." *Lancet* 377: 139–46.

Oreopoulos, Philip, Mark Stabile, Randy Walld, and Leslie L. Roos. 2008. "Short-, Medium-, and Long-Term Consequences of Poor Infant Health: An Analysis Using Siblings and Twins." *Journal of Human Resources* 43 (1): 88–138.

Over, Mead. 2010. "Sustaining and Leveraging AIDS Treatment." Center for Global Development, London.

Peeters, A., L. Bonneux, W. J. Nusselder, C. De Laet, and J. J. Barendregt. 2004. "Adult Obesity and the Burden of Disability Throughout Life." *Obesity Research* 12: 1145–51.

Perkins, Kenneth A., Eric Donny, and Anthony R. Caggiula. 1999. "Sex Differences in Nicotine Effects and Self-Administration: Review of Human and Animal Evidence." *Nicotine and Tobacco Research* 1 (4): 301–15.

Permutt, T., and J. R. Hebel. 1989. "Simultaneous-Equation Estimation in a Clinical Trial of the Effect of Smoking on Birth Weight." *Biometrics* 45 (2): 619–22.

Popkin, Barry M. 2008. "Will China's Nutrition Transition Overwhelm its Health Care System and Slow Economic Growth?" *Health Affairs* 27 (4): 1064–76.

Popkin, Barry M., Susan Horton, Soowon Kim, Ajay Mahal, and Jin Shuigao. 2001. "Trends in Diet, Nutritional Status, and Diet-related Noncommunicable Diseases in China and India: The Economic Costs of the Nutrition Transition." *Nutrition Reviews* 59 (12): 379–90.

Popkin, M. B., S. Kim, E. R. Rusev, S. Du, and C. Zizza. 2006. "Measuring the Full Economic Costs of Diet, Physical Activty and Obesity-Related Chronic Diseases." *Obesity Reviews* 7: 271–93.

Prentice, Andrew M. 2006. "The Emerging Epidemic of Obesity in Developing Countries." *International Journal of Epidemiology* 35 (1): 93–99.

Rao, Vijayendra. 1997. "Wife-Beating in Rural South India: A Qualitative and Econometric Analysis." *Social Science and Medicine* 44 (8): 1169–80.

Rao, Vijayendra, Indrani Gupta, Michael Lokshin, and Smarajit Jana. 2003. "Sex Workers and the Cost of Safe Sex: The Compensating Differential for Condom Use Among Calcutta Prostitutes." *Journal of Development Economics* 71 (2): 585–603.

Rehm, Jürgen, Colin Mathers, Svetlana Popova, Montarat Thavorncharoensap, Yot Teerawattananon, and Jayadeep Patra. 2009. "Global Burden of Disease and Injury and Economic Cost Attributable to Alcohol Use and Alcohol-Use Disorders." *Lancet* 373 (9682): 2223–33.

Robinson, Jonathan, and Ethan Yeh. 2011. "Transactional Sex as a Response to Risk in Western Kenya." *American Economic Journal: Applied Economics* 3 (1): 35–64.

Rooth, Dan-Olof. 2009. "Obesity, Attractiveness, and Differential Treatment in Hiring." *Journal of Human Resources*, 44(3): 710–35.

Ross, Hana, Dang vu Trung, and Vu Xuan Phu. 2007. "The Costs of Smoking in Vietnam: The Case of Inpatient Care." *Tobacco Control* 16 (6): 405–09.

Royer, Heather. 2009. "Separated at Girth: U.S. Twin Estimates of the Effect of Birth Weight." *American Economic Journal: Applied Economics* 1 (1): 49–85.

Sakata, R., P. McGale, E. J. Grant, K. Ozasa, R. Peto, and S. C. Darby. 2012. "Impact of Smoking on Mortality and Life Expectancy in Japanese Smokers: A Prospective Cohort Study." *BMJ Open.*

Thirumurthy, Harsha, Joshua Graff Zivin, and Markus Goldstein. 2008. "The Economic Impact of AIDS Treatment: Labor Supply in Western Kenya." *Journal of Human Resources* 43 (3): 511–52.

Thirumurthy, Harsha, A. Jafri, G. Srinivas, V. Arumugam, R. M. Saravanan, S. K. Angappan, M. Ponnumsamy, S. Raghavan, M. Merson, and S. Kallolikar. 2011. "Two-Year Impacts on Employment and Income Among Adults Receiving Antiretroviral Therapy in Tamil Nadu, India: A Cohort Study." *AIDS* 25 (2): 239–46.

Tsai, S. P., C. P. Wen, S. C. Hu, T. Y. Cheng, and S. J. Huang. 2005. "Workplace Smoking Related Absenteeism and Productivity Costs in Taiwan." *Tobacco Control* 14 (Suppl I): i33–37.

Tucker, Glenn M., and Larry A. Friedman. 1998. "Obesity and Absenteeism: An Epidemiologic Study of 10,825 Employed Adults." *American Journal of Health Promotion* 12 (3): 202–07.

Tumwesigye, Nazarius Mbona, Grace Bantebya Kyomuhendo, Thomas Kennedy Greenfield, and Rhoda K. Wanyenze. 2012. "Problem Drinking and Physical Intimate Partner Violence Against Women: Evidence from a National Survey in Uganda." *BMC Public Health* 12.

UBS. 2012. "Prices and Earnings: A Comparison of Purchasing Power Around the Globe."

UNAIDS (Joint United Nations Programme on HIV/AIDS). 2010. *Global Report: UNAIDS Report on the Global AIDS Epidemic.* New York: UNAIDS. http://www .childinfo.org/files/20101123_GlobalReport_em.pdf.

UNODC (United Nations Office on Drugs and Crime). 2012. *World Drug Report 2012.* Vienna: United Nations.

Wamoyi, Joyce, Daniel Wight, Mary Plummer, Gerry Hiliary Mshana, and David Ross. 2010. "Transactional Sex Amongst Young People in Rural Northern Tanzania: An Ethnography of Young Women's Motivations and Negotiation." *Reproductive Health* 7 (1): 2.

Whitaker, Robert C., Jeffrey A. Wright, Margaret S. Pepe, Kristy D. Seidel, and William H. Dietz. 1997. "Predicting Obesity in Young Adulthood from Childhood and Parental Obesity." *New England Journal of Medicine* 337 (13): 869–73.

WHO (World Health Organization). 2005. *Impact of Tobacco-Related Illnesses in Bangladesh.* Geneva: WHO.

———. 2011. "Global Status Report on Alcohol and Health." WHO, Geneva.

WHO and International Union Against Tuberculosis and Lung Disease. 2007. *A WHO/The Union Monograph on TB and Tobacco Control: Joining Efforts to Control Two Related Global Epidemics.* Geneva: World Health Organization.

World Bank. World Development Indicators. Various years. http://data.worldbank
.org/data-catalog/world-development-indicators.

World Bank and IFC (International Finance Corporation). 2011. *Healthy Partnerships: How Governments Can Engage the Private Sector to Improve Health in Africa.* Washington, DC: World Bank.

Yang, Lian, Hai-Yen Sung, Zhengzhong Mao, Teh-wei Hu, and Keqin Rao. 2011. "Economic Costs Attributable to Smoking in China: Update and an 8-Year Comparison, 2000–2008." *Tobacco Control* 20 (4): 266–72.

Yoon, Kun-Ho, Jin-Hee Lee, Ji-Won Kim, Jae Hyoung Cho, Yoon-Hee Choi, Seung-Hyun Ko, Paul Zimmet, and Ho-Young Son. 2006. "Epidemic Obesity and Type 2 Diabetes in Asia." *Lancet* 368 (9548): 1681–88.

Young, Alwyn. 2005. "The Gift of the Dying: The Tragedy of AIDS and the Welfare of Future African Generations." *Quarterly Journal of Economics* 120 (2): 423–66.

Yusuf, Salim, Steven Hawken, Stephanie Ôunpuu, Leonelo Bautista, Maria Grazia Franzosi, Patrick Commerford, Chim C Lang, Zvonko Rumboldt, Churchill L Onen, Liu Lisheng, Supachai Tanomsup, Paul Wangai Jr, Fahad Razak, Arya M Sharma, Sonia S Anand, on behalf of the INTERHEART Study Investigators and others. 2005. "Obesity and the Risk of Myocardial Infarction in 27000 Participants from 52 Countries: A Case-Control Study." *Lancet* 366 (9497): 1640–49.

Zivin, Joshua Graff, Harsha Thirumurthy, and Markus Goldstein. 2009. "AIDS Treatment and Intrahousehold Resource Allocations: Children's Nutrition and Schooling in Kenya." *Journal of Public Economics* 93 (7/8): 1008–15.

4

Targeting Risky Behaviors Using Nonprice Interventions—Legislation, Information, and Education

Aakanksha H. Pande

Introduction

There is an increasing global prevalence of risky behaviors stemming from the consumption of drugs, alcohol, tobacco, and high-calorie foods, and from engagement in unsafe sex. These behaviors affect individuals' health status and raise their potential to contract communicable diseases like HIV, hepatitis C, and other sexually transmitted infections (STIs). They also increase individuals' risk for developing noncommunicable diseases (NCDs) like diabetes, cardiovascular disease, and certain types of cancers (for example, lung or oral). When multiplied across the population, these diseases result in chronic conditions that have substantial health and monetary effects. Since curtailing these risky behaviors is a public health priority, understanding the evidence behind different types of interventions to curtail them is a public health imperative.

This chapter reviews the global evidence on the effectiveness of nonprice approaches in reducing risky behaviors. It analyzes secondary data on the effectiveness, length of effect, and unintended consequences for each type of intervention. Where possible, it draws on evidence from low- and middle-income countries; however, given the scarcity of such data, it also presents the experiences of high-income countries in tackling risky behaviors. It aims to inform policy makers in developing countries of the choice of interventions to tackle these risky behaviors. Since most nonprice interventions are implemented at a population-level, the chapter may be particularly useful to governments that have the scale, resources, and political commitment to execute them.

What Constitutes a Nonprice Approach to Address Risky Behaviors?

What makes individuals change their behavior? This question has long perplexed economists, psychologists, sociologists, and public health specialists. To answer it, one first needs to understand why individuals participate in risky behaviors, which is addressed in detail in chapter 2. Conventional wisdom suggests that individuals indulge in risky behaviors when they believe that the gain outweighs the harm. This can be due to such factors as time-discounting preferences, incomplete information, or risk-taking propensities among others. To influence changes in behaviors, policy levers must address these flawed heuristics. This is the broad rationale behind the design of all interventions to tackle such behaviors.

In this book, we broadly classify interventions to address risky behaviors using two types of mechanisms—price and nonprice. Price mechanisms primarily use prices and taxation as ways to regulate risky behaviors. This approach tends to be under the purview of economic bodies such as treasuries, commerce departments, and trade organizations. A detailed discussion on price-linked approaches and their impacts on risky behaviors is presented in chapter 5. Nonprice approaches are based on legislation, provisions of substitutes, and information and education campaigns. These population-level interventions are traditionally under the leadership of public health bodies, so they can also be considered "public health approaches." In effect, this is somewhat of an artificial classification, but it is used to improve readability and present interventions suited to different types of policy implementation bodies. Depending on financial and political commitments, the interventions that governments can choose to implement involve differing degrees of involvement, ranging from light to heavy (figure 4.1). Of these options, this chapter reviews the effectiveness of nonprice regulations that include commands and controls, channel factors, voluntary controls, and education and information.

Why Is It Important to Understand the Effects of Nonprice Interventions on Risky Behaviors?

It is important to understand the effects of nonprice interventions on risky behavior for three reasons—if effective, they can lead to millions of lives

Figure 4.1   Range of Interventions Involving Different Degrees of Government Interventions

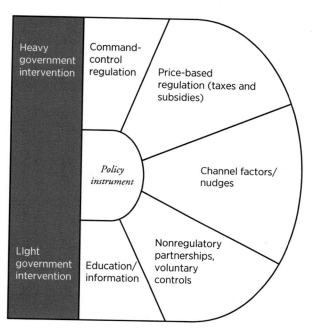

Source: Meiro-Lorenzo, Villafana, and Harrit 2011.

being saved; they often constitute a large portion of public health agencies' budgets; and they can be politically controversial to implement.

The importance of effective interventions to reduce risky behaviors cannot be understated. Behaviors like risky sex and the sharing of needles linked to injecting drug use lead to the spread of communicable diseases like hepatitis C, STIs, and HIV, which are incurable and often fatal. Risky behaviors linked to tobacco use, alcohol consumption, and unhealthy diet fuel the global rise of NCDs such as diabetes, cardiovascular disease, and certain types of cancers as described in chapter 3. This is not a scourge restricted to high-income countries alone. The epidemiological transition is taking place in low- and middle-income countries as they move along the growth trajectory, with increases in death and disability due to NCDs versus communicable diseases worldwide, as discussed in chapter 1.

In an effort to stem the NCD tide, countries are encouraged to reallocate larger sums of money to nonprice interventions for the prevention of risky behaviors (United Nations General Assembly 2012). These reallocations can be in the form of national prevention programs, such as tobacco

BOX 4.1

Nudges as Ways to Encourage Healthful Behaviors

"Nudges" or choice architecture mechanisms are gaining traction as potential ways to encourage consumers to make healthful choices. As described by Oliver (2011), the essence of the approach is to apply behavioral economic insights (for example, loss aversion—losses tend to "hurt" more than gains of the same size) to policy considerations so as to change the environment. For example, people with a tendency to be overweight may place too much emphasis on immediate pleasures at the expense of future harms. In theory, changing the environment will make people more likely to make voluntary decisions that they would like to make and yet ordinarily fail to. The approach involves no compulsion: people are free to engage in the behavior change intervention if they wish and are not required to alter their behavior if they ultimately do not wish to do so. The role of the government is seen as one of an enabler—it can create environments where nudges to encourage more healthful behaviors are present, but it does not enforce the practice of these behaviors.

Despite the field being relatively new, several innovative interventions are being piloted for risky behaviors. These include using smaller glasses to encourage less alcohol consumption, reducing portion sizes of sugar-sweetened beverages to reduce caloric intake, making skim milk the default option instead of full fat milk at coffee shops, and reconfiguring stairwells to be more prominent than elevators, encouraging people to take the stairs.

When evidence is present on the effectiveness of such interventions (such as with the case of calorie labeling in this chapter and the evidence on commitment devices in chapter 5), they have been included in the review. However, for the bulk of such pilots, the evidence on their population-level effectiveness is as yet insufficient. That said, this is a promising field to closely follow, as new methods to encourage healthful behavior may emerge.

Source: Oliver 2011.

cessation programs. These reallocations have two costs—the direct costs of the prevention interventions, and the indirect opportunity costs from not spending that money on other interventions that may have the ability to save more lives.

Given the pervasive and at times socially controversial nature of risky behaviors, interventions to address them can be politically charged. Before diverting scarce health resources and using political currency, it is important for governments to understand the effectiveness of nonprice interventions. For example, governments' decisions to reduce transmission of HIV through the support of needle or syringe exchange programs (NSPs) were extremely controversial. Opponents argued that governments were meant to prevent illegal behaviors, such as use of injecting contrabands, not promote their safe use. Similarly, approaches to restricting the intake of high-calorie foods through "fat taxes" and discussions on bans on large servings of sugar-sweetened beverages have met with dissent. The debate has centered on the role of the government in controlling individual choice, summed up in the refrain—"Will the government now order you to eat broccoli?"

How Is This Chapter Organized?

If risky behaviors can be thought of as the regular consumption of harmful substances or practices (that is, "risky goods" like alcohol, drugs, unhealthy foods, and unsafe sex), then nonprice interventions can be targeted at the two actors involved in every such transaction—producers and consumers. Regardless of behavior, the interventions targeted to each type of actor tend to be similar. Interventions targeted to producers include legislation regulating sales, and interventions targeted to users include information and education campaigns and restrictions on purchasing. By pooling the evidence across different risky behaviors, commonalities emerge that can help guide policy makers in their selection of appropriate interventions (table 4.1).

The chapter is organized according to the target of each intervention. It first reviews evidence for each risky behavior according to interventions targeted at producers, and then it reviews interventions for similar behaviors targeted at consumers. The choice of evidence presented is somewhat purposeful. Preference is given to studies that are based in the developing world that use experimental or quasi-experimental designs to understand the effect of each intervention. However, due to limited data, observational studies with simple difference-in-difference designs are also presented. The potential biases due to unobserved confounding and selection biases are very real concerns; results are to be interpreted with caution. Evidence from these types of studies should be understood as associations at best and not as proof of causality. This prioritization of experimental and quasi-experimental design is similar to the levels of evidence presented in systematic meta-analyses of medical and public health literature like those presented in Cochrane Collaborative Reviews.

A large number of public health interventions to address risky behaviors are being implemented (box 4.1). Due to the limitations of space, this chapter does not aim to present a summary of all of the existing evidence on all interventions, or to present a discussion on the relative costs of their implementation in economic, social, or political terms. To be as useful as possible to policy

Table 4.1 Selection of Interventions to Combat Risky Behaviors

Risky behaviors	Targeted at producers	Targeted at consumers	Prohibition
Illicit drugs	• Cultivation eradication • Law enforcement crackdowns • Crop substitution	• Purchasing restrictions on prescription drugs • Harm reduction programs • Decriminalization of marijuana	• Exists
Tobacco use	• Tobacco industry denormalization • Crop substitution • Trade limits	• Ban on tobacco advertising • Mass media campaigns • Graphic labeling of cigarette packaging including plain packaging • Clean air laws	• Very rare; can include ban on sale of tobacco products, like gutka
Alcohol	• Regulation of alcohol content in beverages	• Ban on advertising • Establishing minimum legal drinking age • Information and education campaigns	• Existed at different points in history and still in some countries
Dietary behaviors leading to obesity	• Restrictions on trans fats	• School-based nutritional education and supplementation programs • Calorie labeling • Restrictions on food advertising to children	
Risky sex	• Criminalization versus decriminalization of sex work • Encouragement of safer sex behaviors among sex workers	• Mass media campaigns • Voluntary counseling and testing • School-based sexual and reproductive health programs	

makers, it prioritizes those interventions that are more recent and that are being actively considered for implementation in low- and middle-income countries. It also strives to cover the different types of interventions being considered—legislation, prohibition, education campaigns—even though it may not review all examples linked to each type. Often, the effects within the type are the same. Where possible, results of meta-analyses or systematic reviews are presented to allow for an overview of all relevant works.

That said, it should be cautioned that the chapter in itself is not a meta-analysis. Due to differences in methodologies, variations across country contexts, differences in types of risky behaviors, and differences in degrees of implementation, the effect sizes of different types of interventions across all studies cannot be pooled. The results are meant to summarize the effectiveness, duration of effect, and potential consequences of non-price interventions being considered to allow policy makers to make informed choices as they confront the increasing incidence of chronic diseases. To this end, the chapter concludes with a pooling of lessons learned, as well as a summary of limitations and areas for future research.

Interventions Targeted at Producers

Interventions targeted at producers primarily consist of enacting and enforcing legislation. These rules can be used to restrict the production of "risky goods," as in the case of drugs and high-calorie food. They can also aim to regulate the production of these goods so as to make them safer, as in the case of the legalization of sex work and mandatory HIV and STI testing of sex workers. The effectiveness of such types of interventions is linked to the enforcement capacity of the government.

Illicit Drugs

Eradication of supply

The supply of illicit drugs can be regulated through the eradication of cultivation. This was enacted on a large scale in Afghanistan. In late 2000 and early 2001, the Taliban government enforced a ban on poppy farming via threats, forced eradication, and public punishment of transgressors. To study the impact of these interventions on poppy cultivation, researchers compared poppy cultivation in Taliban areas with that in non-Taliban areas of Afghanistan, neighboring countries, and non-contiguous comparison areas of Myanmar (Farrell and Thorne 2005). Alternate possible causes of reduction, such as drought, migration, or changes in global opium markets, were reviewed and excluded. The results suggested a 99 percent reduction in the areas of opium poppy farming in Taliban-controlled areas. Globally, this led to a 35 percent reduction in poppy cultivation and a 65 percent reduction in the potential illicit heroin supply from harvests in 2001.

While the intervention could be considered effective in the short run, its effects were seen to diminish when the enforcement mechanisms were reduced. With the subsequent fall of the Taliban, supply of opium once again increased on the global market. Also, the medium- and long-term displacement effects—with other producers increasing supply to match global demand—could not be assessed, as the enforcement mechanisms lasted for a relatively short time. While the intervention was successful in reducing opium supplies, the brutality of enforcement mechanisms can also be questioned. This questionable enforcement process makes it hard to recommend such methods as feasible ways to limit the supply of illicit drugs.

Law enforcement mechanisms

Drug-based law enforcement mechanisms can also have an effect on limiting the supply and subsequently decreasing consumption. This is demonstrated in a study from Australia (Weatherburn and others 2003). From 1998 to 2000, state and federal police in Australia arrested a number of key importers and distributers of heroin and seized large quantities of the drug (almost 750 kilograms in 1999). This resulted in a "heroin drought" at the end of 2000, with an increase in price. Purity, consumption, and expenditure of heroin were reported to have decreased as a result of the shortage, and incidents of fatal heroin overdose also declined significantly. Results suggested that an increase of 1 percent in the price per pure gram of heroin was associated with a decrease of 0.32 percent in expenditures on heroin.

However, this intervention had an unintended consequence—the drop in the availability of heroin was followed by an increase in cocaine use, suggesting a substitution effect. In addition, this study lacked a suitable comparison group and only looked at self-reported changes over time among select drug users (a difference-in-difference test). This introduces several biases into the study design and makes it hard to prove a causal link between reductions in supply and subsequent reductions in consumption.

Crop substitution

Providing farmers with incentives to replace drug crops with other cash crops could potentially be a successful strategy, but only if local realities are taken into account. Bolivia, once heralded as the success story of coca supply reduction, is now witnessing an increase in coca cultivation (Lupu 2004). In 1985, a five-year alternative development program was implemented in the Yungas valley region, which supplies 15 percent of Bolivia's coca production. Communities agreed to not grow coca in return for infrastructure projects, agricultural credits, and a technical package of inputs to help cultivate new varieties of coffee. However, most farmers were not interested in coffee, resulting in only the richest farmers agreeing to the substitution. The project also had the unintentional consequence of the infrastructure projects benefiting drug traffickers.

Tobacco Use

Most tobacco control strategies focus on population-level efforts to decrease the demand for cigarettes through measures that restrict the marketing of tobacco products and encourage individuals to adopt healthier behaviors. However, few interventions have been targeted at tobacco companies and farmers, even though these have met with some success.

Tobacco industry denormalization

Tobacco industry denormalization (TID) includes themes, campaigns, and perspectives developed to combat the process of industry normalization promoted by cigarette manufacturers. It is defined as a public health strategy aimed at "reducing tobacco use by alerting the public to why, despite the fact that tobacco is a legal product, the tobacco industry and its behaviors fall outside the norms of behavior of legitimate businesses" (Mahood 2004). The rationale for TID is captured in the World Health Organization's (WHO) Framework Convention for Tobacco Control (FCTC): "There is a fundamental and irreconcilable conflict between the tobacco industry's interests and public health policy interests" (WHO 2013, 5). TID includes a focus on advocacy, research, and policy.

A recent review of TID interventions suggests that it is an effective population-level tobacco control strategy that contributes to reduced smoking prevalence among youth and young adults, reduces smoking initiation among youth, increases intention to quit, and reduces perceived peer smoking prevalence (Malone, Grundy, and Bero 2012). Evidence is mixed on TID's impact on intentions to smoke, youth empowerment, and views of the industry and its regulation, but studies from California suggest TID's importance as part of comprehensive social norm change programs (Malone, Grundy, and Bero 2012). Given the growing outreach of tobacco companies in new markets in the developing world, TID can be an effective supply-side intervention to combat their influence.

Crop substitution

Crop substitution for tobacco farmers as a way to reduce tobacco yields has met with some success, as demonstrated in Brazil (Vargas and Campos 2005). Strategies to encourage farmers to grow alternatives to tobacco and to diversify their crop portfolio were effective, since the diversification programs were included in a broader development agenda. Farmer organizations played a key role in the organization of the program, and local organizations provided training and technical support to small farmers. The farmers were convinced of the economic sense in shifting production away from tobacco, as the change was associated with higher profitability. However, success was limited because of a considerable contingent of small growers dedicated to tobacco growing, and the economic importance of the activities connected to tobacco production and processing in several municipalities.

Contrasting this with the less successful example of coca substitution in Bolivia (Lupu 2004) suggests that such interventions should be designed and implemented by local bodies to ensure maximum buy-in. Also, providing incentives to all downstream beneficiaries of crop production can increase the probability of long-term impacts.

Limitations on trade
With global reductions in tariff barriers and increases in trade, there is a concern that tariffs on tobacco and tobacco products will also decrease. The FCTC has explicitly addressed this by asking signatory countries to ensure that tariffs on such products are maintained (box 4.2). It is too early to evaluate if this request has been effective.

The illicit trade or smuggling of tobacco products is a serious concern, as it can erode the ability of governments to raise revenues through sin taxes. It has the potential to undermine price and tax measures to strengthen tobacco control, and so result in an increase in the accessibility and affordability of tobacco products for young, poor, and vulnerable persons. According to available estimates, the size of the illicit trade varies in countries from 1 percent to 40–50 percent, 11.6 percent globally, 16.8 percent in low-income countries, and 9.8 percent in high-income countries. The total lost revenue is about US$40.5 billion a year. If this illicit trade were eliminated, governments would gain at least US$31.3 billion a year; from 2030 onward, more than 164,000 premature deaths a year could be avoided, the vast majority in low- and middle-income countries (Joossens and others 2010).

Recognizing this, the Conference of the Parties to the FCTC passed the Protocol to Eliminate Illicit Trade in Tobacco Products at the fifth session in November 2012. Interventions to combat smuggling include harmonizing tax and pricing policies, regulating transport and retail sales, influencing consumers not to purchase smuggled products, and increasing the certainty and severity of punishment through enhanced law enforcement and prosecution mechanisms.

The effects of implementing this protocol by governments is too early to be measured, but it could be useful to curb the supply of tobacco in developing countries. Tajikistan, an FCTC signatory, is one of the first countries to codify this into law by means of a presidential decree that went into effect in January 2013, requiring traders wishing to buy or sell tobacco products to receive special governmental permission.

Excessive Alcohol Use

Regulation of alcohol content
Evidence is lacking on the effectiveness of regulating the alcohol content of beverages on consumption behaviors. As of 2013, India was one of the few known developing countries considering mandating the amount of ethyl alcohol content allowed in distilled spirits, such as whisky, rum, gin, or vodka, as well as for wine and beer, but no rigorous evidence of its impact on health outcomes is available.

Dietary Behaviors Leading to Obesity

Regulating calorie content–trans fat bans

Regulating the calorie content of foods and enforcing the production of healthier food options could potentially be a powerful means to reduce obesity. While this type of regulation of caloric content is yet to be implemented, the only such similar intervention of making foods "healthier" is the banning of trans fats in fast foods in the United States, making it a useful example to study. While trans-fat bans were primarily introduced to reduce the prevalence of cardiovascular disease, simian studies suggest that there may be an independent link between trans fats and obesity (Kavanagh and others 2007). In addition, if unhealthy substances were to be similarly regulated, like the amount of salt or sugar content in packaged foods, it is likely that the effect on taste, preference, and consumption could be similar to that seen through the banning of trans fats.

In 2008, New York City became the first U.S. city to ban restaurants from serving food prepared with partially hydrogenated vegetable oil, or dishes that contain more than 0.5 gram of trans fat per serving. A before-and-after study of consumer choices during this period revealed that diners consumed 2.4 fewer grams of trans fat per lunch after the ban went into effect (Angell and others 2012). The decline was offset by a slight (0.55 gram) increase in consumption of saturated fats, which is associated with elevated cholesterol levels. Diners of all socioeconomic groups shared equally in the benefits.

The authors suggest that reasons for the observed changes in trans-fat content per purchase could include customers selecting a different mix of products, reformulation of menu items, and changes in item size. Inspection of the most commonly purchased food items in chains with the largest reductions in trans fat per purchase (hamburgers, Mexican food, and fried chicken chains) revealed multiple examples of reformulation and new product introductions.

Given the weak pre-post nature of the study design, it would be impossible to attribute changes in trans-fat consumption solely to the ban, but an interesting association is revealed that could be further evaluated through a more rigorous controlled quasi-experimental design.

Risky Sex

Supply-side interventions to reduce risky sexual behavior either crack down on sex work, or they acknowledge its ubiquity and focus on enabling sex workers and high-risk groups to engage in less risky sex through harm-reduction strategies. These strategies include decriminalization, licensing or regulation of sex workers, mandating condom use, and regular STI testing in sex work environments (table 4.2).

Table 4.2 Interventions for Sex Work Harm Reduction

	Initiatives	**Harms reduced**
Education	Peer education, outreach programs, accessible and appropriate materials, sex worker involvement	Drug use, disease, violence, debt, exploitation
Empowerment	Self-esteem, individual control, safe sex, solidarity, personal safety, negotiating skills, refusal to clients, service access, societal acceptance	Drug use, disease, violence, debt, discrimination, exploitation
Prevention	Male and female condoms, lubricants, vaccines, behavioral change, voluntary HIV counseling and testing, participation in research	Drug use, disease
Care	Accessible, acceptable, high-quality, integrated care; prevention-care synergy; prophylaxis; STIs, HIV, and psychological care; social support	Drug use, disease, violence, exploitation
Occupational health and safety	Control of exposure and hazards, treatment for injuries and diseases, employer duties, worker rights	Drug use, disease, violence, debt, exploitation
Decriminalization of sex workers	Sex worker organizations, sex work projects, nongovernmental organizations	Criminalization, discrimination, violence
Rights-based approach	Education, telephone hotlines, training targeted and user-friendly services, government action, media, PREVENT, refugee package, community development	Exploitation (for example, child prostitution, human trafficking, exploitation of mobile populations)

Source: Rekart 2005.

Note: PREVENT = psychological counseling, reproductive health services, education, vaccinations, early detection, nutrition, treatment.

Decriminalization of sex work

Although sex work is illegal in many countries, it is ubiquitous in most. Accordingly, the WHO and several agencies have adopted a more pragmatic approach, urging countries to decriminalize sex work as a means to reduce violence against sex workers and increase access to and availability of health services. Evidence of the effect of decriminalization on health outcomes is limited. Anecdotal evidence from sex workers, clients, and brothel owners in Nevada in the United States (Brents and Hausbeck 2005) and Australia (Seib, Fischer, and Najman 2009) suggests that legalization of sex work decreases violence against sex workers and the transmission of STIs.

Mandating condom use

Mandating condom usage in sex work environments has been another supply-side intervention to make sex work less risky. Thailand's 100 percent condom campaign increased condom use in commercial sex transactions from 14 percent to 94 percent by making condoms freely available, sanctioning noncompliant brothels, and advising men through the media to use condoms with prostitutes (Hanenberg and others 1994). This resulted in a sharp decline in HIV infections. However, recent reports of a significant decline in condom use by brothel-based female sex workers in Thailand underscore the need for such interventions to be sustained in order for effect sizes to be maintained (Buckingham and others 2005; Kerrigan and others 2012).

Interventions Targeted at Consumers

Public health interventions targeted at consumers aim to restrict access to risky goods through legislation like criminalization of drug use and the establishment of minimum legal drinking ages. Interventions may also aim to diminish consumers' desire for these goods through information and education campaigns like calorie labeling laws. They may also work to make the consumption of goods less risky through interventions like condom promotion, decriminalization of less harmful drugs, and needle exchange programs. In general, legislation has been more effective than education programs in restricting risky behaviors, though in the long-run behavior change programs may have more sustained effects.

Illicit Drugs

Needle or syringe exchange programs

A pragmatic public health approach to dealing with drug use has been to promote interventions to reduce adverse health side effects. A cornerstone of such harm reduction approaches has been evident in NSPs for injecting drug use. A recent meta-analysis of 11 NSPs covering 50 percent of the injecting population in low- and middle-income countries suggests their effectiveness in reducing HIV and hepatitis C infection (Des Jarlais and others 2013). The review included high-coverage programs from Bangladesh; Brazil; China; Estonia; Iran; Lithuania; Taiwan, China; Thailand; and Vietnam. In five studies, HIV prevalence in the target population decreased (range −3 percent to −15 percent); in three studies, the hepatitis C prevalence decreased (range −4.2 percent to −10.2 percent). However, in two studies, HIV prevalence increased (range 5.6 percent to 14.8 percent); hepatitis C incidence remained stable in one study. Of the four national reports of newly reported HIV cases, three indicated decreases during NSP expansion, ranging from −30 percent to −93.3 percent, while one national report documented an increase (37.6 percent).

Mandated withdrawal programs like opioid substitution programs

Other interventions target drug users to help them overcome their dependence and include managed withdrawal programs. Such programs, such as opioid substitution programs, aim to reduce the side effects of opioid withdrawal through a tapered substitution of methadone or buprenorphine, which is usually administered orally in a supervised clinical setting. Opioid substitution therapy is endorsed by the Joint United Nations Program on HIV/AIDS, the United Nations Office on Drugs and Crime, and the WHO, and methadone and buprenorphine are on the WHO essential medicines list (Kermode and others 2011). For injecting drug users who also have HIV, such programs have been found to improve adherence to antiretroviral therapy and improve the mental and physical health of participants (Lawrinson and others 2008). These programs attract many injecting drug users who would otherwise have no contact with any health services, suggesting that the programs act as gateways to other services, including primary health care; HIV testing; antiretroviral therapy; and services for tuberculosis, hepatitis C, and STIs. A meta-analysis of 23 controlled trials involving 2,467 adult opioid users in various countries suggests that the slow tapering with temporary substitution of long-acting opioids could reduce withdrawal severity, especially when compared to a placebo group (Amato and others 2013).

Decriminalization of marijuana

Another approach to reduce the effect of illicit drugs on consumers has been to decriminalize the use of less harmful substances, most often marijuana. While politically controversial, the public health impacts are understudied. Where available, data suggest a substitution effect, with users switching from other drugs to marijuana. For example, a study from the United States from 1975–78 suggests that marijuana decriminalization was accompanied by a significant reduction in hospitalization episodes involving illicit drugs other than marijuana, but an increase in marijuana-linked episodes. Although possible biases in study design preclude robust conclusions, the results suggest that some substitution occurs toward the less severely penalized drug when punishments are differentiated (Model 1993).

Another public health effect of decriminalization has been the reduction in non-drug crimes and the violence that often accompanies them, as seen in the United Kingdom (Adda, McConnell, and Rasul 2011). This reduction may be because decriminalization allows police forces to focus their efforts on non-drug crime enforcement, with a consequent decrease observed in these types of crimes. With new laws decriminalizing marijuana in the states of Colorado and Washington in the United States, these effects should be further studied.

Purchasing restrictions on prescription drugs

The explosion of prescription drug abuse in several high-income settings has countries grappling with ways to stem this epidemic. A recent public health intervention in the United States has been to implement prescription restrictions. For example, New York City banned prescriptions of certain painkillers in emergency rooms of public hospitals in 2013. Under the new policy, most public hospital patients will no longer be able to get more than a three-day supply of narcotic painkillers like Vicodin and Percocet. Long-acting painkillers, including OxyContin, a familiar remedy for chronic backache and arthritis, as well as Fentanyl patches and methadone, will not be dispensed at all. Lost, stolen, or destroyed prescriptions will not be refilled. The effect of this intervention is too early to determine, but any evaluation will have to balance the benefits from possible reductions in drug overdoses with negative impacts on pain management.

Tobacco Use

Bans on tobacco advertising

The Framework Convention on Tobacco Control, the world's first global public health treaty, became effective in February 2005 (box 4.2).

The FCTC calls for comprehensive bans on tobacco advertising. However, the effects of advertising bans on tobacco use have been controversial and the evidence mixed. There are perhaps as many studies that show no effect as there are studies that have shown some effect. There is a weak consensus that bans on ads promoting tobacco products and the culture of tobacco use have some effect in high-income countries (Gallet 1999; Nelson 2003, 2006; Saffer and Chaloupka 2000; Schneider, Klein, and Murphy 1981). Where effective, comprehensive bans have been found to be more successful than limited bans. This is consistent regardless of the time period when the bans were implemented—the 1970s or the 1990s—which is noteworthy, given the perceived cultural context of tobacco use.

However, in developing countries, tobacco advertising bans have demonstrated some effect on consumption. A pooled study of advertising bans in 51 countries, including 30 upper-middle-, lower-middle-, and low-income countries, suggests that both comprehensive as well as limited policies are effective in reducing consumption, although comprehensive bans have a far greater impact (Blecher 2008). Limited bans resulted in a 13.6 percent reduction in per capita consumption of tobacco in developing countries, whereas comprehensive bans resulted in a 23.5 percent reduction.

BOX 4.2

What Is the Framework Convention on Tobacco Control?

The Framework Convention on Tobacco Control (FCTC) was signed by 168 of the 192 World Health Organization member states, and more than 170 member states have become parties to the convention. It seeks "to protect present and future generations from the devastating health, social, environmental, and economic consequences of tobacco consumption and exposure to tobacco smoke" by enacting a set of universal standards stating the dangers of tobacco and limiting its use in all forms worldwide. The FCTC provides an internationally coordinated response to combating the tobacco epidemic and identifies specific steps for governments, including supply- and demand- side measures to achieve the following:

- Adopt tax and price measures to reduce tobacco consumption
- Ban tobacco advertising, promotion, and sponsorship
- Create smoke-free work and public spaces
- Put prominent health warnings on tobacco packages
- Combat illicit trade in tobacco products
- Support smoking cessation programs
- Encourage crop substitution
- Ban the sale of tobacco products to minors.

Source: WHO 2003.

Furthermore, advertising bans may be even more effective in the developing world; this is important, given the fact that the fastest number of new tobacco users is in the developing world.

Mass media campaigns

Mass media campaigns using television, radio, newspapers, billboards, posters, leaflets, and booklets can be effective in influencing smoking behavior. They have been found to be most effective in young people under the age of 25 years, especially if the campaign is sustained and intense (Brinn and others 2010; Wilson and others 2012). For example, a time series analysis of a campaign in Australia found that an increase in 1,000 gross rating points (a measure of advertising reach and frequency) led to a reduction in adult smoking prevalence of 0.8 percent within two months, after controlling for price (Wakefield and others 2008). The study also found that the effect dissipated rapidly, suggesting that sustained high levels of exposure are necessary to maximize reductions in smoking prevalence.

Mandating packaging and labeling of tobacco products
Signatory countries to the FCTC have to include graphic warnings and labeling according to specified parameters on tobacco products, such as cigarette boxes. These must be rotating health warnings that cover at least 30 percent of the front and back of boxes. Beyond these minimum requirements, the FCTC states that warnings "should" cover 50 percent or more of a package's principal surfaces and "may" include pictures.

A meta-analysis of 94 studies, mostly from high-income countries, consistently found that the impact of these health warnings depends upon their size and design (Hammond 2011). Obscure text-only warnings appear to have little impact. Prominent health warnings on the face of packages can serve as a major source of health information for smokers and nonsmokers, increase health knowledge and perceptions of risk, and promote smoking cessation. The evidence also indicates that comprehensive warnings are effective among youth and may help to prevent smoking initiation.

Pictorial health warnings that elicit strong emotions, and larger warnings with pictures, are significantly more effective than smaller, text-only messages. Smokers who had read, thought about, and discussed the new labels at baseline were more likely to have quit, made an attempt to quit, or reduced their smoking three months later, after adjusting for intentions to quit and smoking status at baseline (Hammond and others 2003). Evidence from a randomized controlled trial demonstrated that pictorial warnings were associated with a significantly higher motivation to quit. A pictorial warning was also associated with higher fear intensity. The effect of warnings appeared to be independent of nicotine dependence and self-affirmation, suggesting that they may be effective in increasing heavy smokers' motivation to quit (Schneider, Gadinger, and Fischer 2012).

Plain packaging
Australia, with the enactment of the Tobacco Plain Packaging Act in 2011, is the first country to implement "plain packaging" of cigarettes. This refers to packaging that requires the removal of all branding (colors, imagery, corporate logos, and trademarks). The law requires that manufacturers print only the brand name in a stipulated size font and place on the package, in addition to health warnings and any other legally mandated information, such as toxic constituents and tax-paid stamps. The appearance of all tobacco packs is standardized, including the color of the pack.

While the population-level effects of plain packaging have not yet been evaluated, experimental studies exposing select participants to different types of packaging show that plain packaged cigarettes are associated with a less favorable taste and an increased desire to quit. The effect was found to be especially large in youth and women, who are among the fastest growing segments of tobacco users, and may suggest that this is a promising strategy for reducing future smoking rates (Moodie and Ford 2011; Thrasher and others 2011; Wakefield and others 2008).

For example, in one study, 640 Brazilian women ages 16–26 participated in an online survey. Participants were randomized to view 10 cigarette packages according to one of three experimental conditions: standard branded packages, plain packaging, or the same packs without brand imagery or descriptors, such as flavors. Participants rated packages on perceived appeal, taste, health risk, smoothness, and smokers' attributes. Finally, participants were shown a range of branded and plain packs from which they could select a free gift, which constituted a behavioral measure of appeal. The results suggested that branded packs were rated significantly more appealing, better tasting, and smoother on the throat than plain packs. Branded packs were also associated with a greater number of positive smoker attributes, including style and sophistication, and they were perceived as more likely to be smoked by females than the plain packs. Removing descriptors from the plain packs further decreased the ratings of appeal, taste, and smoothness; it also reduced the associations with positive attributes. In the pack offer, participants were three times more likely to select branded packs than plain packs (White and others 2012).

Clean air laws and smoking bans

Several countries have instituted clean air laws. These laws ban smoking in public places, such as bars, restaurants, and buildings. While the evidence is mixed, most studies suggest that implementation of these laws is associated with a 5–10 percent reduction in tobacco consumption (Evans and others 1999; Levy and Friend 2003; Wilson and others 2012; Yurekli and Zhang 2000).

The effectiveness of a smoking ban likely depends on the comprehensiveness of legislation, level of enforcement, public support, degree of prior legislation in place, and length of time that the ban has been in place. For example, Uruguay became the first Latin American country to create 100 percent smoke-free spaces due to the championing of the then-President Dr. Tabaré Vázquez, an oncologist, in 2005. Tobacco consumption within urban areas in Uruguay (home to 95 percent of the population) saw one of the quickest declines in the world. From 2005 to 2011, per-person consumption in Uruguay decreased in relative terms by an estimated 4.3 percent annually (equivalent, with annual compounding, to 23 percent over six years). The biggest drop was recorded in young smokers. The 30-day prevalence of tobacco use in Uruguayan students ages 13 years, 15 years, and 17 years decreased by an estimated 8.0 percent annually, compared with a decrease of 2.5 percent annually in Argentinian students from 2001 to 2009 (Abascal and others 2012).

Smoking bans also lead to a reduction in exposure to passive smoking. A review of 50 studies found that hospitality workers experienced a greater reduction in exposure to secondhand smoke after implementing public bans, compared to the general population (Callinan and others 2010). As a result, smoking bans were associated with improvements in health status in smoking and non-smoking populations, as measured in a reduction in cardiac arrest cases among the general population.

Excessive Alcohol Use

Bans on alcohol advertising

Bans on advertising alcohol have produced mixed results. While some studies suggest a subsequent decline in consumption, they can be critiqued due to potential endogeneity effects. When instrumental variable techniques are used, no effects of advertising bans are seen. For example, a study of bans on broadcast advertising in 17 Organisation for Economic Co-operation and Development (OECD) countries from 1977 to 1995, on per capita alcohol consumption, liver cirrhosis mortality, and motor vehicle fatalities, indicated that advertising bans in these countries have not decreased alcohol consumption or alcohol abuse (Nelson and Young 2001).

Mandating a minimum legal drinking age

A more effective policy to restrict the use of alcohol, especially among minors between the ages of 18 and 21 years, may be the mandating of a minimum legal drinking age. Research from the United States found that the establishment of a minimum age of 21 years versus 18 years was associated with a decrease in the frequency of drinking, as well as a decrease in mortality due to road traffic accidents and suicides. It was calculated that reducing the minimum legal drinking age from 21 years to 18 years would result in eight additional deaths per 100,000 per year in the 18- to 20-year-old age range. However, no effect was seen on the intensity of drinking as measured by number of drinks consumed at a sitting (Carpenter and Dobkin 2011; Miron and Tetelbaum 2009).

A minimum drinking age of 21 years also led to a decrease in maternal drinking prior to birth (Fertig and Watson 2009). This decrease had the additional beneficial cross-generational effect on the health of the fetus, which extends throughout the lifecycle of child. However, these effects should be interpreted with caution, as emerging evidence also suggests a substitution effect, with people switching from alcohol to marijuana use, which may have other deleterious effects (DiNardo and Lemieux 2001).

Information and education campaigns

As with other behavioral change interventions, information and education campaigns on alcohol abuse are shown to have limited effects. For example, a review of 56 studies of educational interventions aimed at primary prevention of alcohol misuse by young people showed limited effect (Foxcroft and others 2003). Only one culturally focused skills training had some protective effect (Schinke, Tepavac, and Cole 2000). This was a school and community intervention with Native American students. A skills-based intervention group that learned cognitive and behavioral skills for substance abuse prevention was approximately and significantly 7 percent less likely than a control group to be weekly drinkers three and a half years after baseline measurement.

Dietary Behaviors Leading to Obesity

Ban on advertising to minors

Advertising of junk food targeted to children has been found to affect children's preferences, purchasing behaviors, and consumption, not only for different brands but also for different food and beverage categories. This effect has been found to be especially strong among children from ages 2 to 11 years (Hastings and others 2006; Institute of Medicine 2006). Evidence from 10 OECD countries found a significant association between the proportion of children overweight and the number of advertisements per hour on children's television, especially those advertisements that encourage the consumption of energy-dense, micronutrient-poor foods (Lobstein and Dibb 2005). In response to this finding, a number of agencies like the Institute of Medicine in 2006 and the WHO in 2004 endorsed marketing practices and policies that acknowledged the vulnerability of children and encouraged marketing practices to promote healthful foods and beverages (Grant and others 2010).

However, translation of these policy positions to action has only been witnessed in a few countries. Sweden and Norway do not allow advertising targeted to children younger than 12 years of age. In Denmark and Belgium, child-directed advertising is significantly restricted. The province of Quebec in Canada banned fast-food advertising to children in television and print in 1978. An evaluation of this intervention showed that fast-food sales declined by an estimated 13 percent, and childhood obesity rates in Quebec were significantly lower than the national average (Dhar and Baylis 2011).

School-based nutritional education and supplementation programs

School-based interventions attempt to change eating habits in formative years and so prevent the downstream effects of poor diet. School-based interventions generally fall into two categories: multicomponent programs that motivate and engage children and families to change their eating behaviors, and single-component programs that provide free or subsidized fruit and vegetables.

A recent meta-analysis of 21 school-based interventions estimated that they improved daily fruit and vegetable consumption by an average of one-quarter to one-third of a portion, equivalent to a 20–30 gram daily increase (Evans and others 2012). Although most schemes aimed to improve the intake of both fruit and vegetables, the schemes failed to increase vegetable intake by a useful amount, with most of the improvement made in fruit intake. The exclusion of fruit juices, which tend to be sugary and not strongly associated with health outcomes, attenuated the impact of these programs. Multicomponent programs tended to result in larger improvements in fruit and vegetable intake than single-component programs, but the limited number of studies within each category precluded robust conclusions from being reached.

The main limitation is that few studies have followed a cohort over time to see if the beneficial effects of such interventions persist. This is an important area for future research.

Calorie labeling

Making consumers aware of the nutritional impacts of their food choices has long been considered as a way to reduce obesity. The most recent set of interventions aims to provide point-of-service information on specific calories being consumed, the hypothesis being that this information will lead consumers to choose lower-calorie options. Labeling the caloric content of foods, either prepackaged or open, is one tool promoted to reduce obesity. While this intervention is still limited to populations in high-income countries—as seen in New York City, New York; San Francisco, California; Multnomah County, Oregon; and King County, Washington—its popularity makes it important to evaluate as a potential intervention to be applied in low- and middle-income countries. The evidence on the impact of calorie and nutritional labeling is mixed. It can be effective in making people more aware of nutrition choices; however, there has been less evidence to suggest that this awareness always translates into selecting more healthful options.

While a number of recent studies has looked at the effect of calorie labeling, many use observational designs, which make it hard to determine causality. One systematic review looked at experimental or quasi-experimental evaluations of the impact of calorie labeling, comparing calorie-labeled menus with no-calorie menus (Swartz, Braxton, and Viera 2011). Only two of the seven studies reported a statistically significant reduction in calories purchased among consumers using calorie-labeled menus, leading the authors to conclude that calorie labeling does not decrease calorie purchasing or consumption. Similarly, a review of point-of-purchase calorie labeling on cafeteria or restaurant food choices shows weak or inconsistent effects (Harnack and French 2008). Given that several of the studies included in this review had methodological limitations, the results should be interpreted with caution.

The mixed message when it comes to effect size could be due to differences in food types studied. An evaluation of the effect of calorie labeling at the Starbucks chain in New York City showed that mandatory calorie posting caused average calories per transaction to decrease by 6 percent, though the effect was due to changes in foods purchased only. Three-quarters of the reduction in calories per transaction was due to consumers buying fewer food items, and one-quarter of the effect was due to consumers substituting lower-calorie items. There was no effect of calorie labeling on the purchase of beverages, the reason most people go to Starbucks, suggesting that effects of calorie labeling may be different depending on consumer taste, preferences, and types of products (Bollinger, Leslie, and Sorensen 2011).

The lack of a consistent effect may also be due to problems in implementation. For calorie labeling to be effective, consumers have to be aware of the existence of labels and then understand their content. Accompanying labels with educational materials has been found to increase awareness and improves selection of healthful choices (Harnack and French 2008). It would be useful to have a more nuanced understanding of the behavioral processes of consumers who stated that "calorie labeling influenced their choice" but who still did not purchase fewer calories. For example, in New York City, 27.7 percent of low-income people who saw calorie labeling said the information influenced their choice, but the evidence did not suggest a detectable difference in calories purchased (Elbel and others 2009).

It can be argued that the scale of the obesity epidemic is so large that even a small change in consumer behavior can have a large impact. For example, a health impact assessment of calorie labeling in Los Angeles County, California, assumed a conservative effect of calorie labeling on food choice. Assuming that if even one in 10 of the restaurant patrons ordered reduced-calorie meals in response to calorie postings, this would still result in an average reduction of 100 calories per meal, and so would avert 40.6 percent of the 6.75 million pound average annual weight gain in the county population ages 5 years and older (Kuo and others 2009).

Risky Sex

Mass media campaigns

Mass media campaigns have often been used to try to change risky sexual behavior. A review of 24 mass media interventions on changing HIV-related knowledge, attitudes, and behaviors showed mixed results, when significant, with a small to moderate effect size (in some cases, increases as low as one to two percentage points) (Bertrand and others 2006). For two of seven outcomes, at least half of the studies showed a positive impact of mass media on the knowledge of HIV transmission and reductions in self-reported, high-risk sexual behavior. Mass media campaigns had little effect on condom use, perceived risk of contracting HIV, interpersonal communication about AIDS or condom use, self-efficacy to negotiate condom use, and abstinence from sexual relations. Studies included had a before-and-after design, a control group, or post-only data over varying levels of exposure. These selection criteria still have threats to internal validity due to historical effects or selection biases, and so they would be considered inadequate to prove causality.

Voluntary counseling and testing

Learning one's HIV status and receiving counseling are not only important steps to receiving care and treatment, they are also important for changing related risk behaviors. A systematic review of 17 studies in low- or middle-income countries found that voluntary counseling and testing for HIV are effective in reducing some HIV-related risk behaviors, including decreasing the number of self-reported sexual partners of participants (Fonner and others 2012). Condom use was also significantly increased among participants who tested HIV-positive during voluntary counseling and testing, but no effect on condom use was seen when results were pooled across sero status.

School-based interventions

School-based sexual and reproductive health programs have been associated with changes in self-reported teenage sexual behavior. A global review of self-reported sexual behavior in the aftermath of HIV education programs showed that two-thirds of programs reported a delay in sexual debut or an increase in condom use (Kirby, Laris, and Rolleri 2007). At least 10 interventions were found to have long-term behavioral impacts lasting two or more years after the intervention. Most evaluations of school sex education programs show them to be associated with an increase in self-reported knowledge and attitudes regarding sexuality, pregnancy, and contraception. However, it was not always clear if this increased knowledge led to changes in behavior (DeLamater, Wagstaff, and Havens 2000; Eggleston and others 2000; Gallant and Maticka-Tyndale 2004; Speizer, Magnani, and Colvin 2003).

When self-reported data are replaced with biological endpoints, the results are somewhat tempered. The few randomized studies of school-based interventions that use biological endpoints suggest a more limited role of general school-based interventions. A randomized trial of training teachers in the Kenyan government's HIV education curriculum showed no real impact on teen pregnancy, a biological endpoint for change in sexual behavior (Duflo and others 2006). However, when education programs included more targeted messages, changes in biological endpoints were seen. In another Kenyan study, providing information on the relative risk of HIV infection by partner's age led to a 28 percent decrease in teen pregnancy, an objective proxy for the incidence of unprotected sex (Dupas 2011). In contrast, the official abstinence-only HIV curriculum had no impact on teen pregnancy.

The contrasting results highlight the need to interpret self-reported sexual behavior change data, such as the number of sexual partners or the use of condoms, with utmost caution. Self-reported sexual behavior data have been documented to be very unreliable markers of actual sexual behavior, with the direction of the bias hard to predict (Phillips and others 2010; Roberts and others 1996). Of even more concern is that often the direction of bias can be correlated to the intervention itself. For example, if an intervention is an education program that encourages reducing sexual partners, due to a social desirability bias participants may be more likely to report reducing the number of sexual partners, even if this is not actually the case.

When self-reported data are triangulated with biological data, results often diverge. For example, a study of the STI consequences of adolescent virginity pledges in schools in the United States showed that while pledgees reported abstaining from sex, rates of sexually transmitted diseases did not differ between pledgees and non-pledgees (Brückner and Bearman 2005). Until biological data are used as endpoints of such studies, it will be challenging to gain conclusive evidence on the impact of such programs on risky sexual behavior. Correlations between increases in information and education campaign coverage and declines in HIV prevalence are available from several African countries, including Uganda and Zimbabwe. However, without more rigorous evidence drawn from robust experimental or quasi-experimental studies grounded in biological endpoints, it is challenging to infer causality.

Prohibition

Prohibition is defined as the absolute and total ban on producing or consuming a substance that applies to all members of society. It has been used with illicit drugs, alcohol, and tobacco in selected instances.

Illicit Drugs

While prohibition can be successful in severely limiting the legal market for a product, it can often lead to the creation of a flourishing black market, promote corruption, and result in a substitution effect among contraband substances (Miron 2003; Miron and Zwiebel 1995). This was seen in the increase in heroin use in Asia due to the anti-opium laws implemented in the 1960s (Westermeyer 1976). However, the restriction in the legal market also led to an increase in the prices of narcotics, which is assumed to have decreased opium consumption.

Tobacco Use

Bhutan is the only country to completely outlaw the cultivation, harvesting, production, and sale of tobacco and tobacco products under the Tobacco Control Act of Bhutan 2010. It is too early to evaluate the effectiveness of this law; given the political opposition that had to be navigated to secure its passage, it may provide useful lessons to other countries.

In India, gutka, a highly addictive carcinogenic chewing product containing a mixture of betel nut, tobacco, slaked lime, and flavorings, has been banned in 24 states and three union territories as of May 2013. Anecdotal evidence suggests that enforcement has been problematic, with small shopkeepers not displaying the product openly but selling it if requested. Evidence is unavailable on the effectiveness of this ban on health conditions, such as oral cancers.

Excessive Alcohol Use

Perhaps the best-known public health intervention to abolish supply of a risky good has been the prohibition of alcohol. Prohibition is in effect in several countries or subregions presently due to religious beliefs, as in Islamic countries, or sociocultural beliefs, as in the state of Gujarat in India. To study the effects of prohibition on alcohol use, it is useful to look at countries that went through limited periods of prohibition and compare the use before, during, and after these laws. Two examples are from prohibition in the United States in the 1920s and in India in the 1990s.

Three rigorous studies use interrupted time series methods to look at the effects of prohibition in the United States as a result of the 18th Amendment to the U.S. Constitution in 1920 (Dills, Jacobson, and Miron 2005; Dills and Miron 2004; Miron and Zwiebel 1991). All studies reported a sharp decline in alcohol consumption during Prohibition to almost 30 percent of the pre-Prohibition level. This resulted in a reduction in cirrhosis by 10 to 20 percent and in arrests by 20 to 30 percent during the period. When prohibition was initially lifted, the effects persisted in the short term. However, in the subsequent decade, alcohol consumption increased sharply to 60 to 70 percent of its pre-Prohibition level.

Similar effects were seen in India during periods of complete and partial prohibition introduced in different states in India since Independence in 1947 (Rahman 2009). Prohibition in India was of different types—complete prohibition of all alcohol items and partial prohibition of certain types of local alcohol only, like arrack. This allowed the effect of prohibition on different types of alcohol to be studied and showed that it was successful in reducing the consumption of different types of alcohol, with a greater effect in urban households.

Conclusions and Lessons

Looking across the different risky behaviors, common themes emerge in terms of types of public health interventions that tend to be effective, enabling conditions, duration of effects, and negative externalities.

What Types of Interventions Are Most Likely to Be Effective?

The review looks at the effectiveness of two broad types of nonprice interventions—legislation, and information education and communication programs—on changing risky behaviors. In terms of effectiveness, the evidence suggests that legislation tends to be more effective, especially if enforcement mechanisms are strong. For example, comprehensive advertising bans on cigarettes were found to be more effective than partial advertising bans. Similarly, the prohibitions of alcohol in America and poppy cultivation in Afghanistan were both stringently enforced; the results were sharp decreases in use of both substances. That said, the mechanisms of enforcement are not always condoned, as seen in the case of the Taliban in Afghanistan, and perhaps due to the strict policing, the unintended consequences of these policies were especially severe. In reality, enforcing watertight restrictions is often extremely challenging, especially in countries with a weak state capacity for enforcement.

In general, information and education campaign programs have been found to be less effective in changing behavior. Calorie labeling laws and school-based sex education programs are effective in informing consumers about the risks associated with certain behaviors. But translating that knowledge into concrete and consistent changes in behavior seems to be harder to achieve.

This is not meant to discredit all information and education efforts as ineffective—far from it. As the case of graphic warnings on cigarettes has shown, messages that are targeted and reinforced at regular intervals can be very effective in changing behavior. It can also be the case that information and education campaigns work to influence general societal attitudes toward risk, and they are accordingly harder to measure, making it more challenging to prove effectiveness. Information and education campaigns are certain to play a very important role in changing attitudes and must go hand-in-hand with any risky behavior change programs.

What Is the Duration of the Effect, If Any?

In terms of length of effects, it can be argued that the opposite may be true—behavior change programs may be more effective in the long run than legislation. For example, if changing consumer preferences results in alterations in demand, this dynamic may have longer-lasting effects in reducing risky behaviors than by constraining supply, since demand often bounces back when supply returns. As demonstrated, changing consumer behavior over a prolonged period is challenging and may require a combination of interventions and incentives. Multidisciplinary research on these questions is under way, and the results of such studies will be very useful to better understanding the most effective mix of interventions to foster more healthful preferences.

The review of the evidence suggest that even if an intervention is effective, the duration that the effect is maintained varies, and it is a function of the length and intensity with which the intervention is delivered. When the intervention is removed, there is likely to be a "bounce back" effect to levels similar to those before the intervention. This was seen in the case of the removal of prohibition in the United States and the fall of the Taliban in Afghanistan. In both cases, within a few years, alcohol consumption increased to pre-Prohibition levels, and poppy cultivation increased to pre-Taliban levels.

Even if an intervention is maintained for a long time, its effect may be attenuated. For example, Thailand's 100 percent condom law has been found to be less effective now than immediately after its passage. This decrease in condom use is attributed to a possible desensitization, coupled with changing perceptions of HIV risk going from an incurable disease to a chronic condition. To prevent a similar desensitization, the FCTC requires that graphic warnings on cigarette boxes be rotating so that smokers are continually exposed to new images, which will reinforce the message.

What Are the Enabling Conditions for Interventions to Be Effective?

Across risky behaviors, certain enabling conditions emerge that make it more likely for interventions to be effective. These conditions involve the design, targeting, and implementation of the interventions.

In terms of design of the intervention, interventions found to be more successful take into account local culture. This is seen by comparing the success of Brazil's tobacco substitution program to that of Bolivia's coca program. The former involved the community in the choice of the substitute crop and method of farming, while the latter was imposed on the community.

Targeting interventions to subpopulations is also important—simply because an intervention is not effective in a general population does not necessarily imply that it will not be effective in a subset. For example, voluntary counseling and testing is found to be more effective in changing behavior among subpopulations who test positive for HIV. Similarly, mass media campaigns for tobacco use are found to be more effective in youth, and tobacco advertising bans may be more effective in developing countries.

In terms of the implementation of the intervention, legislation supported by a strong enforcement mechanism tends to be more effective. This is seen in the success of stringently enforced clean air laws in reducing tobacco use and associated morbidity and mortality. Similarly, repeated messaging is effective, as with the case of graphic labeling on cigarette packages that reinforce the message to smokers each time they reach for a cigarette.

What Are the Possible Negative Effects, If Any?

An important lesson that emerges from this review is that even when interventions are effective, externalities often emerge that need to be considered. This is especially the case when a substance is banned, as substitution effects tend to take place. These can be negative, as when opium bans result in an increase in heroin use. They can also be beneficial, as when the legalization of marijuana resulted in not only a decrease in the rate of overdose of heroin and opium due to people switching to marijuana, but also a decrease in violent crime, partially due to local police forces being freed up from enforcing marijuana-related crackdowns.

Before implementation, policy makers need to think through all the potential effects that can result if the intervention is effective, and then try and preempt the negative consequences to the greatest extent possible. At the very least, negative externalities should be assumed and included in the cost-benefit calculus before deciding to implement an intervention.

What Are Future Areas for Research?

In reviewing the effects of public health interventions on risky behaviors, gaps emerge that future researchers should address.

More types of interventions should be considered, or interventions should be extended to different subpopulations. For example, most interventions to reduce tobacco use are targeted to cigarette smokers. This is especially worrisome in the developing world, where alternate forms of tobacco are used including *beedis* and chewing tobacco. These products are often used, by populations who tend to be poorer, and so are already disadvantaged when it comes to diagnosing and treating the illnesses caused by these substances. Similar analogies extend to the lack of interventions targeted to consumers of moonshine and home-brewed alcohol, which can be more lethal due to its unregulated nature.

In addition, there are some glaring gaps where few nonprice interventions are being pioneered. For example, there is a lack of nonprice interventions targeted to producers of high-calorie food. Possibly due to political and economic clout, the food industry has largely escaped legislation and regulation of caloric content. The one intervention covered in this chapter, the banning of trans fats, is believed to have a positive impact on cardiovascular disease suggesting potential beneficial effects from more similar regulation.

In terms of research design, there is an urgent need for more rigorous experimental and quasi-experimental evaluations of health interventions to be undertaken. Most evaluations consist of post-only designs or at best a pre-post design without a control group. This compromises the internal validity of the study and makes it hard to determine the causal effect. Including a suitable control group would greatly strengthen the level of evidence and can often be done easily if considered in the design stage. Staggering the rollout of an intervention, collecting data in adjacent districts to where the intervention is being implemented, or using matching techniques such as propensity score methods can all be helpful ways of creating a suitable counterfactual.

In terms of the geographic spread of evidence, a gap exists in evidence emerging from low- and middle-income countries. This gap is often because interventions are only being introduced in high-income countries, which prevents evaluation results from being available. However, prioritizing evaluations from the start would allow the collection of baseline data and the selection of controls, which would enable rigorous evaluations to be conducted at later stages. With low- and middle-income countries about to experience an increase in noncommunicable diseases, it is even more imperative that robust evidence on effective interventions be generated.

In summary, the results of this review illustrate that effective interventions do exist to tackle risky behavior. If carefully selected and adapted to the local context, it is possible for low- and middle-income countries to successfully protect their populations' health and prevent noncommunicable diseases from developing.

References

Abascal, Winston, Elba Esteves, Beatriz Goja, Franco González Mora, Ana Lorenzo, Amanda Sica, Patricia Triunfo, and Jeffrey E. Harris. 2012. "Tobacco Control Campaign in Uruguay: A Population-Based Trend Analysis." *Lancet* 380 (9853): 1575–82.

Adda, Jérôme, Brendon McConnell, and Imran Rasul. 2011. "Crime and Depenalization of Cannabis Possession: Evidence from a Policing Experiment." Working paper, University College London, U.K.

Amato, Laura, Marina Davoli, Silvia Minozzi, Eliana Ferroni, Robert Ali, and Marcia Ferri. 2013. "Methadone at Tapered Doses for the Management of Opioid Withdrawal." Cochrane Database of Systematic Reviews Online (2) CD003409.

Angell, Sonia Y., Laura K. Cobb, Christine J. Curtis, Kevin J. Konty, and Lynn D. Silver. 2012. "Change in Trans Fatty Acid Content of Fast-Food Purchases Associated with New York City's Restaurant Regulation: A Pre–Post Study." *Annals of Internal Medicine* 157 (2): 81–86.

Bertrand, Jane T., Kevin O'Reilly, Julie Denison, Rebecca Anhang, and Michael Sweat. 2006. "Systematic Review of the Effectiveness of Mass Communication Programs to Change HIV/AIDS-Related Behaviors in Developing Countries." *Health Education Research* 21 (4): 567–97.

Blecher, Evan. 2008. "The Impact of Tobacco Advertising Bans on Consumption in Developing Countries." *Journal of Health Economics* 27 (4): 930–42.

Bollinger, Bryan, Phillip Leslie, and Alan Sorensen. 2011. "Calorie Posting in Chain Restaurants." *American Economic Journal: Economic Policy* 3 (1): 91–128.

Brents, Barbara G., and Kathryn Hausbeck. 2005. "Violence and Legalized Brothel Prostitution in Nevada Examining Safety, Risk, and Prostitution Policy." *Journal of Interpersonal Violence* 20 (3): 270–95.

Brinn, Malcolm P., Kristin V. Carson, Adrian J. Esterman, Anne B. Chang, and Brian J. Smith. 2010. "Mass Media Interventions for Preventing Smoking in Young People." Cochrane Database of Systematic Reviews (11) CD001006.

Brückner, Hannah, and Peter Bearman. 2005. "After the Promise: The STD Consequences of Adolescent Virginity Pledges." *Journal of Adolescent Health* 36 (4): 271–78.

Buckingham, Robert W., John Moraros, Yelena Bird, Edward Meister, and Natalie C. Webb. 2005. "Factors Associated with Condom Use among Brothel-Based Female Sex Workers in Thailand." *AIDS Care* 17 (5): 640–47.

Callinan, Joanne E., Anna Clarke, Kirsten Doherty, and Cecily Kelleher. 2010. "Legislative Smoking Bans for Reducing Secondhand Smoke Exposure, Smoking Prevalence and Tobacco Consumption." Cochrane Database of Systematic Reviews (4) CD005992.

Carpenter, Christopher, and Carlos Dobkin. 2011. "The Minimum Legal Drinking Age and Public Health." *Journal of Economic Perspectives* 25 (2): 133–56.

DeLamater, John, David A. Wagstaff, and Kayt Klein Havens. 2000. "The Impact of a Culturally Appropriate STD/AIDS Education Intervention on Black Male Adolescents' Sexual and Condom Use Behavior." *Health Education and Behavior* 27 (4): 454–70.

Des Jarlais, Don C., Jonathan P. Feelemyer, Shilpa N. Modi, Abu Abdul-Quader, and Holly Hagan. 2013. "High Coverage Needle/Syringe Programs for People Who Inject Drugs in Low and Middle Income Countries: A Systematic Review." *BMC Public Health* 13 (1): 53.

Dhar, Tirtha, and Kathy Baylis. 2011. "Fast-Food Consumption and the Ban on Advertising Targeting Children: The Quebec Experience." *Journal of Marketing Research* 48 (5): 799–813.

Dills, Angela K., Mireille Jacobson, and Jeffery A. Miron. 2005. "The Effect of Alcohol Prohibition on Alcohol Consumption: Evidence from Drunkenness Arrests." *Economics Letters* 86: 279–84.

Dills, Angela K., and Jeffery A. Miron. 2004. "Alcohol Prohibition and Cirrhosis." *American Law and Economics Review* 6 (2): 285–318.

DiNardo, John, and Thomas Lemieux. 2001. "Alcohol, Marijuana, and American Youth: The Unintended Consequences of Government Regulation." *Journal of Health Economics* 20 (6): 991–1010.

Duflo, Esther, Pascaline Dupas, Michael Kremer, and Samuel Sinei. 2006. "Education and HIV/AIDS Prevention: Evidence from a Randomized Evaluation in Western Kenya." Policy Research Working Paper 4024, World Bank, Washington, DC.

Dupas, Pascaline. 2011. "Do Teenagers Respond to HIV Risk Information? Evidence from a Field Experiment in Kenya." *American Economic Journal: Applied Economics* 3 (1): 1–34.

Eggleston, Elizabeth, Jean Jackson, Wesley Rountree, and Zhiying Pan. 2000. "Evaluation of a Sexuality Education Program for Young Adolescents in Jamaica." *Revista Panamericana de Salud Pública* 7 (2): 102–12.

Elbel, Brian, Rogan Kersh, Victoria L. Brescoll, and L. Beth Dixon. 2009. "Calorie Labeling and Food Choices: A First Look at the Effects on Low-Income People in New York City." *Health Affairs* 28 (6): 1110–21.

Evans, Charlotte E. L., Meaghan S. Christian, Christine L. Cleghorn, Darren C. Greenwood, and Janet E. Cade. 2012. "Systematic Review and Meta-Analysis of School-Based Interventions to Improve Daily Fruit and Vegetable Intake in Children Aged 5 to 12 Years." *American Journal of Clinical Nutrition* 96 (4): 889–901.

Evans, William N., Matthew C. Farrelly, and Edward Montgomery. 1999. "Do Workplace Smoking Bans Reduce Smoking?" *American Economic Review* 89 (4): 728–47.

Farrell, Graham, and John Thorne. 2005. "Where Have All the Flowers Gone? Evaluation of the Taliban Crackdown against Opium Poppy Cultivation in Afghanistan." *International Journal of Drug Policy* 16 (2): 81–91.

Fertig, Angela R., and Tara Watson. 2009. "Minimum Drinking Age Laws and Infant Health Outcomes. *Journal of Health Economics* 28 (3): 737–47.

Fonner, Virginia A., Julie Denison, Caitlin E. Kennedy, Kevin O'Reilly, and Michael Sweat. 2012. "Voluntary Counseling and Testing (VCT) for Changing HIV-Related Risk Behavior in Developing Countries." Cochrane Database of Systematic Reviews (9) CD001224.

Foxcroft, David R., Diana Ireland, Deborah J. Lister-Sharp, Geoffrey Lowe, and Rosie Breen. 2003. "Longer-Term Primary Prevention for Alcohol Misuse in Young People: A Systematic Review." *Addiction* 98 (4): 397.

Gallant, Melanie, and Eleanor Maticka-Tyndale. 2004. "School-Based HIV Prevention Programmes for African Youth." *Social Science and Medicine* 58 (7): 1337–51.

Gallet, Craig A., 1999. "The Effect of the 1971 Advertising Ban on Behavior in the Cigarette Industry." *Managerial and Decision Economics* 20 (6): 299–303.

Grant, Robert M., Javier R. Lama, Peter L. Anderson, Vanessa McMahan, Albert Y. Liu, Lorena Vargas, Pedro Goicochea, Martin Casapía, Juan Vincente Guanira-Carranza, Maria E. Ramirez-Cardich, Orlando Montoya-Herrera, Telmo Fernández, Valdilea G. Veloso, Susan P. Buchbinder, Suwat Chariyalertsak, Mauro Schechter, Linda-Gail Bekker, Kenneth H. Mayer, Esper G. Kallás, K. Rivet Amico, Kathleen Mulligan, Lane R. Bushman, Robert J. Hance, Carmela Ganoza, Patricia Defechereux, Brian Postle, Furong Wang, J. Jeff McConnell, Jia-Hua Zheng, Jeanny Lee, James F. Rooney, Howard S. Jaffe, Ana I. Martinez, David N. Burns, and David V. Glidden. 2010. "Preexposure Chemoprophylaxis for HIV Prevention in Men Who Have Sex with Men." *New England Journal of Medicine* 363 (27): 2587–99.

Hammond, David. 2011. "Health Warning Messages on Tobacco Products: A Review." *Tobacco Control* 20 (3): 327–37.

Hammond, David, Geoffrey T. Fong, Paul W. McDonald, Roy Cameron, and K. Stephen Brown. 2003. "Impact of the Graphic Canadian Warning Labels on Adult Smoking Behaviour." *Tobacco Control* 12 (4): 391–95.

Hanenberg, Robert S., Wiwat Rojanapithayakorn, Prayura Kunasol, and David C. Sokal. 1994. "Impact of Thailand's HIV-Control Programme as Indicated by the Decline of Sexually Transmitted Diseases." *Lancet* 344 (8917): 243–45.

Harnack, Lisa J., and Simone A. French. 2008. "Effect of Point-of-Purchase Calorie Labeling on Restaurant and Cafeteria Food Choices: A Review of the Literature." *International Journal of Behavioral Nutrition and Physical Activity* 5 (1): 51.

Hastings, Gerard, Laura McDermott, Kathryn Angus, Martine Stead, and Stephen Thomson. 2006. "The Extent, Nature and Effects of Food Promotion to Children: A Review of the Evidence." Technical Paper, World Health Organization, Geneva.

Institute of Medicine. 2006. "Food Marketing to Children and Youth: Threat or Opportunity?" Consensus Report, Institute of Medicine of the National Academies, Washington, DC.

Joossens, Luk, David Merriman, Hana Ross, and Martin Raw. 2010. "The Impact of Eliminating the Global Illicit Cigarette Trade on Health and Revenue." *Addiction* 105 (9): 1640–49.

Kavanagh, Kylie, Kate L. Jones, Janet Sawyer, Kathryn Kelley, J. Jeffrey Carr, Janice D. Wagner, and Lawrence L. Rudel. 2007. "Trans Fat Diet Induces Abdominal Obesity and Changes in Insulin Sensitivity in Monkeys." *Obesity* 15 (7): 1675–84.

Kermode, Michelle, Nick A. Crofts, M. Suresh Kumar, and Jimmy Dorabjee. 2011. "Opioid Substitution Therapy in Resource-Poor Settings." *Bulletin of the World Health Organization* 89 (4): 243.

Kerrigan, Deanna, Andrea Wirtz, Stefan Baral, N'Della N'Jie, Anderson Stanciole, Jenny Butler, Robert Oelrichs, and Chris Beyer. 2012. *The Global HIV Epidemics among Sex Workers*. Washington, DC: World Bank.

Kirby, Douglas B., B. A. Laris, and Lori A. Rolleri. 2007. "Sex and HIV Education Programs: Their Impact on Sexual Behaviors of Young People throughout the World." *Journal of Adolescent Health* 40 (3): 206–17.

Kuo, Tony, Christopher J. Jarosz, Paul Simon, and Jonathan E. Fielding. 2009. "Menu Labeling as a Potential Strategy for Combating the Obesity Epidemic: A Health Impact Assessment." *American Journal of Public Health* 99 (9): 1680–86.

Lawrinson, Peter, Robert Ali, Aumphornpun Buavirat, Sithisat Chiamwongpaet, Sergey Dvoryak, Boguslaw Habrat, Shi Jie, Ratna Mardiati, Azarakhsh Mokri, Jacek Moskalewicz, David Newcombe, Vladimir Poznyak, Emilis Subata, Ambrose Uchtenhagen, Diah S. Utami, Robyn Vial, and Chengzheng Zhao. 2008. "Key Findings from the WHO Collaborative Study on Substitution Therapy for Opioid Dependence and HIV/AIDS." *Addiction* 103 (9): 1484–92.

Levy, David T., and Karen B. Friend. 2003. "The Effects of Clean Indoor Air Laws: What Do We Know and What Do We Need to Know?" *Health Education Research* 18 (5): 592–609.

Lobstein, Tim, and Sandra Dibb. 2005. "Evidence of a Possible Link Between Obesogenic Food Advertising and Child Overweight." *Obesity Review* 6 (6): 203–08.

Lupu, Noam. 2004. "Towards a New Articulation of Alternative Development: Lessons from Coca Supply Reduction in Bolivia." *Development Policy Review* 22 (4): 405–21.

Mahood, Garfield. 2004. "Tobacco Industry Denormalization: Telling the Truth about the Tobacco Industry's Role in the Tobacco Epidemic." Brochure, Non-Smokers' Rights Association, Toronto.

Malone, Ruth E., Quinn Grundy, and Lisa A. Bero. 2012. "Tobacco Industry Denormalisation as a Tobacco Control Intervention: A Review." *Tobacco Control* 21 (2): 162–70.

Meiro-Lorenzo, Montserrat, Tonya L. Villafana, and Margaret N. Harrit. 2011. "Effective Responses to Non-Communicable Diseases: Embracing Action beyond the Health Sector." Human Nutrition and Population Discussion Paper, World Bank, Washington, DC.

Miron, Jeffrey A. 2003. "The Effect of Drug Prohibition on Drug Prices: Evidence from the Markets for Cocaine and Heroin." *Review of Economics and Statistics* 85 (3): 522–30.

Miron, Jeffrey A., and Elina Tetelbaum. 2009. "Does the Minimum Legal Drinking Age Save Lives?" *Economic Inquiry* 47 (2): 317–36.

Miron, Jeffrey A., and Jeffrey Zwiebel. 1991. "Alcohol Consumption during Prohibition." *American Economic Review* 81 (2): 242–47.

———. 1995. "The Economic Case Against Drug Prohibition." *Journal of Economic Perspectives* 9 (4): 175–92.

Model, Karyn E. 1993. "The Effect of Marijuana Decriminalization on Hospital Emergency Room Drug Episodes: 1975–1978." *Journal of the American Statistics Association* 88 (423): 737–47.

Moodie, Crawford, and Allison Ford. 2011. "Young Adult Smokers' Perceptions of Cigarette Pack Innovation, Pack Colour and Plain Packaging. *Australasian Marketing Journal* 19 (3): 174–180.

Nelson, Jon P. 2003. "Cigarette Demand, Structural Change, and Advertising Bans: International Evidence, 1970–1995." *Journal of Economic Analysis and Policy* 2 (1): 1–29.

———. 2006. "Cigarette Advertising Regulation: A Meta-Analysis." *International Review of Law and Economics* 26 (2): 195–226.

Nelson, Jon P., and Douglas J. Young. 2001. "Do Advertising Bans Work? An International Comparison." Working Paper 6-01-1, Department of Economics, Pennsylvania State University, University Park.

Oliver, Adam. 2011. "Is Nudge an Effective Public Health Strategy to Tackle Obesity? Yes." *British Medical Journal* 342 (apr13-5): d2168–d2168.

Phillips, Anna E., Gabriella B. Gomez, Marie-Claude Boily, and Geoffrey P. Garnett. 2010. "A Systematic Review and Meta-Analysis of Quantitative Interviewing Tools to Investigate Self-Reported HIV and STI Associated Behaviours in Low- and Middle-Income Countries." *International Journal of Epidemiology* 39 (6): 1541–55.

Rahman, Lupin. 2009. "Alcohol Prohibition and Addictive Consumption in India." Working Paper, London School of Economics, London.

Rekart, Michael L. 2005. "Sex-Work Harm Reduction." *Lancet* 366 (9503): 2123–34.

Roberts, Rosebud O., Erik J. Bergstralh, Luanne Schmidt, and Steven J. Jacobsen. 1996. "Comparison of Self-Reported and Medical Record Health Care Utilization Measures." *Journal of Clinical Epidemiology* 49 (9): 989–95.

Saffer, Henry, and Frank Chaloupka. 2000. "The Effect of Tobacco Advertising Bans on Tobacco Consumption." *Journal of Health Economics* 19 (6): 1117–37.

Schinke, Steven P., Lela Tepavac, and Kristin C. Cole. 2000. "Preventing Substance Use among Native American Youth: Three-Year Results." *Addictive Behavior* 25 (3): 387–97.

Schneider, Lynne, Benjamin Klein, and Kevin M. Murphy. 1981. "Governmental Regulation of Cigarette Health Information." *Journal of Law and Economics* 24 (3): 575–612.

Schneider, Sven, Michael Gadinger, and Andreas Fischer. 2012. "Does the Effect Go Up in Smoke? A Randomized Controlled Trial of Pictorial Warnings on Cigarette Packaging." *Patient Education and Counseling* 86 (1): 77–83.

Seib, Charlotte, Jane Fischer, and Jackob M. Najman. 2009. "The Health of Female Sex Workers from Three Industry Sectors in Queensland, Australia." *Social Science and Medicine* 68 (3): 473–78.

Speizer, Ilene S., Robert J. Magnani, and Charlotte E. Colvin. 2003. "The Effectiveness of Adolescent Reproductive Health Interventions in Developing Countries: A Review of the Evidence." *Journal of Adolescent Health* 33 (5): 324–48.

Swartz, Jonas J., Danielle Braxton, and Anthony J. Viera. 2011. "Calorie Menu Labeling on Quick-Service Restaurant Menus: An Updated Systematic Review of the Literature." *International Journal of Behavioral Nutrition and Physical Activity* 8: 135.

Thrasher, James F., Matthew C. Rousu, David Hammond, Ashley Navarro, Jay R. Corrigan. 2011. "Estimating the Impact of Pictorial Health Warnings and 'Plain' Cigarette Packaging: Evidence from Experimental Auctions among Adult Smokers in the United States." *Health Policy* 102 (1): 41–48.

United Nations General Assembly. 2012. "Political Declaration of the High-Level Meeting of the General Assembly on the Prevention and Control of Non-Communicable Diseases." United Nations, New York.

Vargas, Marco Antonion, and Renato Ramos Campos. 2005. "Crop Substitution and Diversification Strategies: Empirical Evidence from Selected Brazilian Municipalities." Health Nutrition and Population Discussion Paper 28, World Bank, Washington, DC.

Wakefield, Melanie A., Sarah Durkin, Matthew J. Spittal, Mohammad Siahpush, Michelle Scollo, Julie A. Simpson, Simon Chapman, Victoria White, and David Hill. 2008. "Impact of Tobacco Control Policies and Mass Media Campaigns on Monthly Adult Smoking Prevalence." *American Journal of Public Health* 98 (8): 1443–50.

Weatherburn, Don, Craig Jones, Karen Freeman, and Toni Makkai. 2003. "Supply Control and Harm Reduction: Lessons from the Australian Heroin 'Drought'." *Addiction* 98 (1): 83–91.

Westermeyer, Joseph. 1976. "The Pro-Heroin Effects of Anti-Opium Laws in Asia." *Archives of General Psychiatry* 33 (9): 1135–39.

White, Christine M., David Hammond, James F. Thrasher, and Geoffrey T. Fong. 2012. "The Potential Impact of Plain Packaging of Cigarette Products among Brazilian Young Women: An Experimental Study." *BMC Public Health* 12: 737.

WHO (World Health Organization). 2003. "WHO Framework Convention on Tobacco Control." WHO, Geneva. http://whqlibdoc.who.int/publications /2003/9241591013.pdf.

————. 2013. "Guidelines for Implementation of the WHO Framework Convention on Tobacco Control." http://apps.who.int/iris/bitstr eam/10665/80510/1/9789241505185_eng.pdf.

Wilson, Lisa M., Erika Avila Tang, Geetanjali Chander, Heidi E. Hutton, Olaide A. Odelola, Jessica L. Elf, Brandy M. Heckman-Stoddard, Eric B. Bass, Emily A. Little, Elisabeth B. Haberl, and Benjamin J. Apelberg. 2012. "Impact of Tobacco Control Interventions on Smoking Initiation, Cessation, and Prevalence: A Systematic Review." *Journal of Environmental and Public Health* 2012: art. 961724.

Yurekli, Ayda A., and Ping Zhang. 2000. "The Impact of Clean Indoor-Air Laws and Cigarette Smuggling on Demand for Cigarettes: An Empirical Model." *Health Economics* 9 (2): 159–70.

5

Using Economic Mechanisms to Reduce Risky Behaviors: Tax Policies and Other Incentives

Damien de Walque

Introduction

Chapter 4 focuses on the effectiveness of information and communication campaigns and regulations, including prohibitions; this chapter discusses prevention interventions based on economic mechanisms, such as prices, taxes, and subsidies and other economic incentives. While this distinction between the two categories of interventions is useful, we acknowledge that it is somewhat arbitrary. For example, drug prohibition is a regulation intervention, but the prohibition decision and the degree of law enforcement that accompany it are likely to have an impact on prices.

The countries in the developed world have used taxes as a mechanism to reduce risky behaviors, such as alcohol and smoking, by increasing their price to consumers. Several developing countries are considering the introduction or increase of taxes on these products. This chapter reviews past and present experiences, with the stated limitation that most of the evidence currently available comes from developed countries. Subsidies have also been used, perhaps less frequently, to encourage safer behaviors. Examples include the distribution of free or subsidized condoms, or the provision of family planning services. In addition to functioning as price interventions, incentives are proposed as a mechanism to discourage risky behaviors or to encourage safe behaviors. Demand-side interventions using financial incentives such as conditional cash transfers (CCTs) have been explored as ways to incentivize safe sex and reduce the prevalence of sexually transmitted infections (STIs). This chapter first investigates the effects of price and tax policy, covering each of the risky behaviors in turn, and then explores other incentive mechanisms, such as CCTs, contingency management, and commitment devices. Contingency management relies on the mechanism of conditionality to elicit behaviors that are viewed to be in one's long-term interests and to discourage behaviors that may be detrimental to one's own health and well-being.

Prices and Taxes

The most basic principle of economics, the law of demand, posits that as the price of a good rises, the demand for that good falls. This principle underlies government policies both to increase revenues and to penalize the use of unhealthy substances. In countries like China, Greece, and Nepal, which have a high prevalence of smoking, a tobacco tax can constitute from 5 percent to 10 percent of total tax revenues (Chaloupka and others 2000).

One reasonable question is whether tax increases are passed to consumers as price increases. Chaloupka and others (2000) address this question in the context of tobacco taxation. They conclude that increases in tobacco taxes, because of the addictive nature of consumption and because of the oligopolistic structure of the industry, will lead to increases in the prices of tobacco products that are likely to match or exceed the increase in the tax in most countries. They further observe that larger increases in prices will occur when there is less potential for cross-border shopping.

We now turn to each of the five risky behaviors covered in this book and review the evidence on how tax policy has affected consumption. An important concept in this discussion is price elasticity, that is, the percentage change in quantity demanded in response to a 1 percent change in price. Given the law of demand, price elasticities are almost always negative. One important consideration, however, is that some harmful products are substitutes for one another. As a consequence, substitution effects can be observed as consumers switch from one type of product to another in response to tax and price changes. This is more likely to occur within a class of product (for example, switching from spirits to wine), or from one type of unhealthy food to another, than across product class (for example, from alcohol to tobacco).

Taxation of Drugs

Because abused drugs are usually illicit, governments cannot directly influence drug prices through taxes. However, the degree of law enforcement, discussed in chapter 4, is a key determinant in drug prices. By varying the severity of the law enforcement, governments can indirectly modify economic incentives to consume illicit drugs as well as influence the type of drugs that are less likely to be consumed. One study has explicitly tried to measure the price elasticity of cocaine and marijuana in the United States (DeSimone and Farrelly 2003). They analyze adults (ages 18 to 39) and youth (ages 12 to 17) from 1990 to 1997. Finding accurate price data for illegal drugs is problematic: they use cocaine prices collected by undercover drug agents, primarily from the Drug Enforcement Administration, and construct a marijuana price estimate from prices listed in the Illegal Drug Price/Purity Report. Their results suggest that adults seem more price sensitive than youth. Adult cocaine demand is negatively related to cocaine price (elasticity of −0.41), but adult marijuana demand is not significantly related to its own price. Cocaine and marijuana prices have limited impact on youth demand for these drugs. The authors speculate that this might be due to a decreased perceived risk and an increased glamorization of drug use among youth, among other reasons. Interestingly, increases in arrest probability diminish both types of drug use.

Taxation of Tobacco

In their review of tobacco taxation in developing countries, Chaloupka and others (2000) conclude that increases in cigarette and other tobacco taxes will significantly reduce both the prevalence of smoking and the consumption of tobacco products. They review a large group of studies. Each study has potential limitations, but taken together, the following picture emerges: most estimates for the price elasticity of demand from the large literature on high-income countries fall into the relatively narrow range from −0.25 to −0.50, with many clustering around −0.40.[1] Gallet and List (2003) conduct a literature review of studies—mainly of high-income countries—from a methodological angle; they conclude that the estimation method has a limited impact on the measured elasticity. Estimates from the much smaller literature on low- and middle-income countries suggest that demand in these countries is more responsive to price than demand in high-income countries, with most estimates in the range from −0.50 to −1.00. This difference in relative price sensitivity is consistent with standard economic theory that suggests that price sensitivity will be greater among those with lower incomes, as well as with the economic theories of addictive behavior that suggest that less educated, lower-income persons will be more responsive to changes in monetary prices than those with more education and higher incomes. Chaloupka and others (2000) further estimate that a global cigarette tax increase that raised prices by 10 percent would reduce premature deaths attributable to smoking by approximately 10 million in the current cohort of smokers, and that almost 90 percent of these extended lives would be for individuals in low- and middle-income countries.

Impact of tax increases on smoking rates
Because of addiction, the impact of tax hikes in reducing smoking is larger in the long run than in the short run. Since the 2000 review by Chaloupka and others, studies have focused on the impact of tobacco taxation in developing countries. In Bangladesh, Zulfiqar, Rahman, and Rahman (2003) estimate that a 10 percent increase in the real price of tobacco leaf decreases consumption by 5.8 percent. Using data from Bangladesh, India, Indonesia, Nepal, Sri Lanka, and Thailand, Guindon, Perucic, and Boisclair (2003) analyze how annual per capita tobacco or cigarette consumption varies with price. They use both a conventional demand model, in which tobacco consumption is a function of the price of cigarettes and real income, and a myopic addiction demand model, in which tobacco consumption also depends on past consumption (one-year lagged consumption). The myopic consumption model predicts that price increases will have a larger impact in the long run than in the short run, because addiction makes consumption less likely to vary or be more "sticky" and dependent on past consumption patterns. In the presence of addiction, the demand in the short run is likely to be more inelastic (that is, an elasticity closer to zero) than in the long run. People addicted to a substance will tend to keep buying it, even when the price increases, at least for a while, hence, the short-run elasticity. However, when they realize the price rise is permanent, they will be more likely to adjust their consumption over time, hence, long-run elasticity.

For all countries, higher prices are associated with lower tobacco consumption. The estimation using the conventional model yields price elasticities ranging from about −0.60 to −0.90, while the myopic addiction models yields short-run elasticities ranging from −0.10 to −0.65 and long-run elasticities from −0.80 to −1.40. Lance and others (2004) analyze the price elasticities of cigarettes in China (data from 1993 to 1997) and Russia (data from 1996 to 2000). Their results indicate that overall price elasticity estimates in China and Russia range from 0 to −0.15. Those estimates are quite small compared to previous studies. However, the high level of consumption suggests a strong addiction of consumers. Moreover, those elasticities may be not relevant for large increases in prices, such as those recently experienced in high-income countries. For China, Hu and others (2010) adopt a different approach: they assume two different levels of price elasticities (−0.15 and −0.50); from those parameters, they estimate the additional tax revenue for the government, the reduction in cigarette consumption, and the number of lives saved. Hidayat and Thabrany (2010) also employ a myopic addiction model to estimate the price elasticity of cigarette smoking, using three waves of the Indonesian Family Life Survey (1993, 1997, and 2000). Their estimates suggest that a 10 percent increase in cigarette prices would lead to a 2.8 percent decrease in cigarette consumption in the short run and a 7.3 percent decrease in the long run (short-run elasticity of −0.28 and long-run elasticity of −0.73).

Impact of tax increases on health outcomes
While most studies of tobacco taxation focus on its impact on consumption, a few go further and look at the impact on health outcomes. Moore (1996) estimates that a 10 percent increase in the tobacco tax will result in a 1.5 percent decrease in respiratory cancer mortality and a 0.5 percent decrease in cardiovascular disease (CVD) mortality. Given a population of 250 million, and at the 1990 annual rate of about 60 respiratory cancer deaths and 400 deaths due to CVD per 100,000, this implies a saving of 2,250 lives from cancer and 4,635 lives from CVD per year. Because reducing respiratory cancer and CVD mortality is the main goal of tobacco control policies, these types of estimates are relevant. However, they also warrant some caution, since many factors could influence death rates, such as medical progress. It might also be more precise to give estimates in terms of life-years saved. Evans and Ringel (1999) and Levy and Meara (2006) examine the impact of cigarette taxes and prices in the United States on prenatal maternal smoking. The results suggest that smoking participation among pregnant women declines as cigarette prices rise. Further, Evans and Ringel (1999) find that average birth weights rise when tobacco excise taxes are increased.

Finally, Gruber and Mullainathan (2005) measure the effect of taxes on tobacco on self-reported happiness in the United States and Canada. They estimate that in the United States, a US$1 rise in cigarette taxes reduces unhappiness of those with a propensity to smoke by roughly 2.5 percentage points, relative to those unlikely to smoke. The authors argue that smokers value cigarette taxation as a self-control device. They compare this variation with a change in income: moving from the bottom to the third income quartile reduces unhappiness by about 4 percentage points. So a US$1.60 tax increase would be equivalent to moving someone with a propensity to smoke from the bottom to the third income quartile. However, when they replicate their analysis with data from Canada, they find effects of smaller magnitude: the estimates imply that a Can $1 tax increase would reduce unhappiness by 0.6 percentage points. Even though they acknowledge that there might be happy smokers, Gruber and Mullainathan (2005) conclude that smokers themselves may be made better off by cigarette taxes, because they have time-inconsistent preferences; in the short run, they prefer smoking, but in the long run, they would like to stop. Higher taxes help them to do what they ultimately want to do, which is smoke less. They use subjective well-being measures, which are interesting but also complicated since the implicit assumption is that individuals share the same definition of happiness and this definition is constant over time.

It is beyond the scope of this book to discuss how tobacco taxation income can be best used, for example, earmarking it for public health programs versus general revenue support. However, it is worth mentioning that even though general revenue support offers more flexibility to the government, earmarking it for public health initiatives might make tobacco taxation more politically acceptable.

Taxation of Alcohol

Tax increases on alcohol lead to a decline in consumption, but the effect varies by type of drink and group of individuals. The literature on alcohol taxation is primarily focused on developed countries (Chaloupka, Grossman, and Saffer 2002; Booth and others 2008), with a few exceptions from developing countries that we will highlight. The literature from developed countries highlights the fact that price elasticities vary by product and that substitution effects can be observed with consumers switching from one type of drink to another in response to tax and price changes (Gruenewald and others 2006; Müller and others 2010; Ramful and Zhao 2008). Many studies also stress that there are different price elasticities for different groups of individuals. For example, in the United States, the evidence is mixed on whether heavy drinkers are more responsive to tax increases (Manning, Blumberg, and Moulton 1995; Nelson 2008; Williams, Chaloupka, and Wechsler 2005). This question of responsiveness by type of drinker is particularly relevant for alcohol, since moderate alcohol consumption may not necessarily represent a significant health risk, but heavy drinking is the main public health concern.

Standard economic theory assumes that tax changes are passed on to the consumer in equivalent price changes. This is a conservative estimate, since empirical work suggests that a 10 percent tax increase will usually generate a price increase of 10 percent to 20 percent, an estimate similar to the one for tobacco taxes (Kenkel 2005; Young and Bielinska-Kwapisz 2006). Among the 91 studies included in Wagenaar, Salois, and Komro (2009), 74 found a significant negative relationship between taxation or prices and consumption, with an overall elasticity estimate of −0.51. Mean elasticities for specific beverages were −0.46 for beer (105 studies), −0.69 for wine (93 studies), and −0.80 for spirits (103 studies). Significant effects were also found for alcohol prices on heavy drinking, although the effect sizes were smaller than for overall drinking (Wagenaar, Salois, and Komro 2009).

Wagenaar's estimates are quite similar to those from another recently published analysis (Gallet 2007), which reported median price elasticities for wine (−0.70), spirits (−0.68), and all alcoholic beverages (−0.50), but a slightly lower price elasticity for beer (−0.36). Gallet (2007) included over 1,000 estimates from studies conducted since 1945. Overall, the demand for beer, wine, and spirits is generally price-inelastic (that is, the price elasticity is between 0 and −1), with the demand for wines and distilled spirits more responsive to prices than the demand for beer. This difference in responsiveness suggests that beer might be part of the usual consumer basket and consumers might find it more difficult to dispense with it.

No specific evidence was identified on effects of price or taxation on those with low incomes. A tax increase sufficient to reduce physical and other consequences of drinking may improve the nation's health. But it might also reduce the available income of drinkers who continue to regularly consume alcohol, since evidence from the meta-analyses of price elasticities suggests that alcohol has considerable price inelasticity.

Effects on youth

Results indicate that youth are particularly sensitive to price increases, but the tax effect on heavy drinkers is smaller than among regular drinkers. The literature also studies the implications of tax increases for population groups that are deemed important for policy. Kuo and others (2003) demonstrate that younger people (ages 15–29) are particularly likely to be affected by price. This result seems to be in contrast with what has been found about the responsiveness of youth to tobacco tax increases. Youth may be especially sensitive to price because they often have little money of their own—but this would be true for cigarette smoking as well. One difference with tobacco might be that young people who drink heavily may not yet be addicted, or may not be so addicted that they become less responsive to price changes. A recent study in the United Kingdom found a strong relationship between teenagers' disposable income and their likelihood to engage in binge drinking (Bellis and others 2007).

The evidence on the impact of alcohol taxation on heavy or problem drinkers of all ages is mixed. Chaloupka and Laixuthai (1997) looked specifically at how price would affect heavy drinking. Given a model of addiction, it is reasonable to suppose that heaviest drinkers will be least affected by price changes. However, some studies have found that heavy drinkers may be more affected by increased prices than moderate or occasional drinkers. This could be explained, at least in part, by the idea that when consuming large quantities as a necessity, a small price increase has a larger effect, but when drinking occasionally as a luxury, the price is less important. The study found that raising beer prices through taxation would cut both the overall number of young drinkers and the number of those who drink heavily. In their meta-analysis, however, Wagenaar, Salois, and Komro (2009) found that price and/or tax increases significantly affect heavy drinking ($p < 0.01$), but that the magnitude of effects is smaller than for the effects on overall drinking.

Impact of tax increases on health outcomes

Taxes on alcohol also have a positive impact on health outcomes, including reduced motor vehicle fatalities. As for tobacco, some studies go beyond the impacts of tax increases on consumption to look at the impact on health outcomes. Saffer and Grossman (1987) first examined the impact of beer excise taxes on youth fatality rates from motor vehicle crashes in the United States. They concluded that increases in beer taxes would significantly reduce youth motor vehicle fatalities. For example, the study predicted that a policy adjusting the beer tax for the inflation rate since 1951 would have reduced fatalities among 18- to 20-year-old youths by 15 percent. Chaloupka, Saffer, and Grossman (1993) and Ruhm (1996) extended and updated this research by considering the effects of beer taxes for more recent periods; they concluded that higher beer excise taxes are among the most effective means for reducing drinking and driving in all segments of the population.

Excessive alcohol consumption can have numerous other adverse health effects; accordingly, reductions in consumption related to price increases might also reduce these adverse health effects. Several studies have examined the impact of alcohol prices on liver cirrhosis mortality rates, a key adverse outcome associated with long-term heavy alcohol consumption that accounts for a large number of deaths annually. For example, Cook and Tauchen (1982) and Grossman (1993) concluded that increases in the excise taxes on alcohol would significantly reduce deaths from liver cirrhosis in the United States, even though Sloan, Reilly, and Schenzler (1994) did not come to the same conclusion. But Sloan, Reilly, and Schenzler (1994) concluded that increases in the price of alcoholic beverages would reduce suicides and deaths from diseases for which alcohol is a contributing factor, but not deaths that are primarily related to alcohol. Ohsfeldt and Morrisey (1997) also examined the impact of alcohol price and availability on injuries, specifically, nonfatal workplace injuries; they found a strong inverse relationship between workplace injuries and beer taxes.

Impact of tax increases in developing countries

The literature studying the effects of alcohol taxation in developing countries is much more limited. Bird and Wallace (2010) document that taxes on alcohol contribute substantially to total tax revenues in many African countries. Okello (2001) analyzes the structure of excise taxation in Kenya and investigates the extent to which the taxes have met their commonly stated objectives, that is, to raise substantial government revenue and to discourage consumption. That study finds that the demand for beer is inelastic to price in the short run but elastic in the long run, with the exception of Guinness beer, which is price-elastic both in the short run and in the long run. Treisman (2010) examines the price regulation of vodka in Russia between 1990 and 2007. He finds that retail sales of both vodka and beer decreased when their prices were high. During periods of intensive price regulation motivated by populism (in 1991 through early 1992) the relative price of vodka fell sharply, and consumption increased.

Taxation of Unhealthy Foods

Taxes on unhealthy foods are a fairly recent phenomenon, and the evidence is more limited, especially from developing countries. Three recent literature reviews focus on the links among food prices, taxes, and obesity. Powell and Chaloupka (2009) review 196 articles; they find limited evidence that weight outcomes could be improved by using fiscal policies, and they conclude that substantial price changes are needed to improve these outcomes significantly. Faulkner and others (2011) conclude that the evidence supports the existence of an effect of food prices on weight outcomes, but that those price effects are small. However, they consider several factors that might contribute to underestimating those effects:

- Current data lack large variation in prices necessary to help identify meaningful effects on people's weight.
- Prices might be endogenous, that is, themselves influenced by other factors.
- Weight and price data might be measured with error, because they are usually self-reported.
- Weight does not increase linearly, and so a repeated small short-term impact could have important long-run consequences.

Mytton, Clarke, and Rayner (2012) advocate taxes on unhealthy foods, but they conclude the tax needs to be at least 20 percent to have a significant impact on health. A recent attempt by Denmark to tax fat food products increased prices by 9 percent. That attempt failed, in part because of cross-border shopping by consumers. Other studies in the United States estimate effects of price or tax increases on food consumption, which are insignificant or small.[2]

These limited impacts of taxes on unhealthy foods on weight might be due to the fact that food products have many substitutes; when a tax is levied on one unhealthy food, consumers can easily switch to another product. Chouinard and others (2007) and Fletcher, Frisvold, and Tefft (2010a, 2010b) estimate that tax increases on dairy products and soft drinks, respectively, would have a small impact in the United States. However, a recent study from Brazil (Claro and others 2012) has estimated larger price elasticities: they found a price elasticity of beverages of −0.85 and an income elasticity of 0.41. The price elasticity was higher (−1.03) for the poor than for the non-poor (−0.63), suggesting that a 1 percent increase in the price of sugar-sweetened drinks would lead to an average decrease in consumption of 0.85 percent (1.03 percent and 0.63 percent for the poor and non-poor, respectively). Ng, Zhai, and Popkin (2008) study the impact of oil prices on dietary composition in China between 1991 and 2000, a period during which the average daily intake of edible oil increased from 23 to 33 grams over nine years, representing a 5 percent increase in the diet composition. They conclude that price policies can affect the dietary composition, among poor people in particular.

Impact of tax increases on unhealthy foods

In contrast with the findings for tobacco and alcohol, the evidence on the impact of taxes on unhealthy food consumption and on obesity is less developed and points overall to smaller effects. This might be because experiments with taxes on that type of food are limited and recent, whereas the literature on tobacco and alcohol taxes is well established and relies on a long history of tax variations. However, more fundamental reasons might explain this contrast. People need to eat to survive, while they can abstain from tobacco and alcohol without health consequences. Many unhealthy foods are inexpensive, while healthier foods are more expensive and require more time for shopping and cooking (cheap doughnut compared to expensive broccoli, for example), as mentioned by Gelbach, Klick, and Stratmann (2009). Differentiated taxes could modify relative prices, but the broad range of healthy and unhealthy foods makes it difficult to avoid substitution among unhealthy foods.

Taxation of Risky Sex

Risky sex is a behavior for which prevention usually involves information and regulation rather than tax levies. However, several studies have documented the responsiveness of sexual behavior to prices, such as sex workers willing to forgo condoms when clients pay additional charges (Gertler, Shah, and Bertozzi 2005; Rao and others 2003). In a commercial sex transaction, the sex worker and the client negotiate the price; the characteristics of the sex worker, such as her attractiveness, might influence the price. Gertler, Shah, and Bertozzi (2005) are able to isolate the premium paid by clients for not using condoms from other factors like attractiveness by using several transactions with and without condoms by the same sex worker.

Other Incentives

Prices and tax increases are direct ways to affect the consumption of unhealthy goods. But while tobacco and alcohol taxation are widespread, other behaviors, such as risky sex or illicit drug use, are difficult to tax since they are not easily observed. Although a tax increase directly raises the price of the risky product, other incentives can financially encourage the safe behavior, indirectly raising the opportunity cost of the risky behavior. Among these incentives are conditional cash transfers (CCTs), contingency management, and commitment devices, as well as loans and subsidies. Given the limited evidence available, we do not discuss those incentive mechanisms behavior by behavior, but rather by type of incentives. These types of incentives might also serve as a nudge, that is, "a soft push" steering people toward better decisions by presenting choices differently, and address the issues of bounded rationality discussed in chapter 2.

Conditional Cash Transfers

CCTs have become an increasingly popular approach for incentivizing socially desirable behavioral change. The principle of conditionality— making payments contingent, for example, on a minimal level of schooling attendance or preventive care use—distinguishes CCTs from more traditional means-tested social programs. The evaluation of CCTs has shown that they can be effective at raising consumption, education, and preventive health care (Lagarde, Haines, and Palmer 2007), as well as actual health outcomes (Fernald, Gertler, and Neufeld 2008; Gertler 2004).

Conditional cash transfers and HIV prevention
The evidence on the efficacy of conditional cash transfers for STI or HIV prevention is still unfolding and remains limited. In Malawi, small financial incentives have been shown to increase the uptake of HIV testing and counseling (Thornton 2008). Another study in Malawi conducted a CCT for adolescents in which the cash transfer was conditional on school attendance; in addition to increased enrollment and attendance, the program also caused a reduction in HIV and HSV-2 (herpes simplex virus–type 2, the common cause of genital herpes) incidence (Baird and others 2012). At follow-up, the HIV prevalence among program beneficiaries was 60 percent lower than the control group (1.2 percent versus 3.0 percent). Similarly, the prevalence of HSV-2 was more than 75 percent lower in the combined treatment group (0.7 percent versus 3.0 percent). No significant differences were detected between those offered conditional and unconditional payments. In addition, cash payments offered to the girls who had already dropped out of school at the beginning of the trial made no

difference to their risk of HIV or HSV-2 infection. The same program also led to a modification of self-reported sexual behaviors, with adolescent girls having younger partners (Baird and others 2010).

To date, two studies evaluated conditional cash transfers in which the condition is attached to negative test results for STIs. In Malawi, Kohler and Thornton (2011) tested an intervention promising a single cash reward in one year's time for individuals who remained HIV negative. This design had no measurable effect on the HIV status, but the number of sero conversions in the sample was very small and statistical power was therefore low.

The RESPECT study (de Walque and others 2012) evaluated a randomized intervention that used economic incentives to reduce risky sexual behavior among young people ages 18–30 and their spouses in rural Tanzania. The goal was to prevent HIV and other STIs by linking cash rewards to negative STI test results assessed every four months. The study tested the hypothesis that a system of rapid feedback and positive reinforcement using cash as a primary incentive to reduce risky sexual behavior could be used to promote safer sexual activity among young people who are at high risk of HIV infection. Results of the randomized controlled trial after one year showed a significant reduction in STI incidence in the group that was eligible for the US$20 quarterly payments, but no such reduction was found for the group receiving the US$10 quarterly payments. Further, while the impact of the CCTs did not differ between males and females, the impact was larger among poorer households and in rural areas.

While the results from those studies are important in showing that financial incentives can be a useful tool for preventing HIV/STI transmission, this approach needs to be replicated and implemented on a larger scale before it could be concluded that such CCT programs, for which administrative and laboratory capacity requirements are significant, offer an efficient, scalable, and sustainable prevention strategy. An ongoing study in Mexico City is testing the use of conditional cash transfers for HIV prevention among men who have sex with men and male sex workers (Galárraga and others 2013). Another ongoing study in Lesotho tests the use of lottery tickets as financial incentives for HIV prevention; preliminary results indicate that the intervention has led to reductions in the rate of new infections among women (Björkman-Nyqvist and others 2013). A lottery design might allow the scaling up of this type of intervention in a cheaper way, since less cash needs to be paid and not all participants would necessarily need to be tested.

Financial incentives for weight loss

Financial incentives have also been tested for weight loss, mainly in developed countries, with mixed results. In an experiment in the United States, financial incentives have been tested to encourage weight loss (Finkelstein and others 2007). The study tests the ability of two levels of modest financial incentives to encourage weight loss among overweight employees in North Carolina. The study design included weight and height measurements and randomly allocated the participants to three groups. After three months, participants with no financial incentives lost two pounds, those receiving US$7 per percentage point of weight lost reduced their weight by approximately three pounds, and those receiving US$14 lost 4.7 pounds. After six months, the financial gains were equalized across the three groups; no statistically significant difference was observed.

In another experiment in the United States, Cawley and Price (2011) find that cash rewards were not successful in leading to weight loss; however, bonds that were only refunded upon successful achievement of year-end weight loss goals led to modest reductions in weight, suggesting that commitment devices might be more effective. Interestingly, however, in Mexico, the Progresa/Opportunidades CCTs, where the cash transfers are not linked to weight loss but to children's school attendance and mothers' attendance at meetings focused on children's health, have been associated with higher body mass index and blood pressure in adults, suggesting that the increased income might have led to an increase in unhealthy food consumption (Fernald, Gertler, and Hou 2008).

Contingency Management Approaches

Similar to CCTs, contingency management (CM) relies on the mechanism of conditionality to elicit behaviors viewed to be in the long-term interests of individuals or society, and to discourage those behaviors that may be ultimately detrimental to individuals' health and well-being that may not be easily perceived or experienced in the short term.

Several key differences between CCTs and CM are summarized in table 5.1.

- First, CCT programs typically have much larger cash rewards for complying with conditionality; hence they exploit both price and income effects on behavior.
- Second, CCT programs have typically conditioned based on easily monitored input behaviors, such as health care use. CM has been used for behaviors, such as drug use, that are harder to monitor directly; consequently, CM conditions based on the desired outcome, for example, a negative drug test result.
- Third, while the CCT-incentivized inputs, such as a prenatal care visit, require a simple behavioral response over which the individual has a high degree of control, CM incentives often require a complex behavioral change over which the individual may have imperfect control (Kane and others 2004). This complexity may require changing multiple

Table 5.1 Comparison between Conditional Cash Transfers and Contingency Management

Similarities

Mechanism	Use conditionality to elicit behaviors that are viewed to be in one's long-term interests, and to discourage behaviors that may have detrimental consequences to one's own health and well-being that may not be easily perceived or experienced in the short term

Differences

	Conditional cash transfers	Contingency management
Amount	Much larger cash rewards for complying with conditionality, exploiting both price and income effects on behavior	Smaller cash rewards, especially as a fraction of average income per capita; often test different amounts
Type of incentives	Usually cash	Cash, but also vouchers or lottery prizes
Type of behaviors conditioned upon	Typically conditioned on easily monitored input behaviors, such as health care use	Used for behaviors hard to directly monitor (such as drug use), and hence conditions instead on the desired outcome, for example, a negative drug test or weight loss
Complexity of behavioral response	Incentivized inputs, for example, a prenatal care visit, require a simple behavioral response over which individual has high degree of control	Incentives often require a complex behavioral change over which the individual may have imperfect control
Targeting	Most frequently based on poverty	Most frequently based on risky behavior
Scale	Some programs on a very large scale	Often on a small, experimental scale
Location	More frequent in developing countries	Mainly in developed countries

Sources: de Walque and others 2012; Medlin and de Walque 2008.

behaviors, reversing habit formation and addictive behaviors, and judging uncertainty, such as the probability that a behavior will indeed cause a negative test.

CM applications span many areas of risky behaviors, including substance abuse, smoking, and overeating. In general, however, they have primarily been implemented and tested in developed countries. They have been especially well studied by clinical psychologists as a therapeutic approach to encourage the practice of healthful behaviors and to discourage unhealthy behavioral practices, especially those that may be linked to addiction or other destructive behaviors that are deeply ingrained or habit-forming. CM interventions provide "reinforcers," for example, incentives or rewards contingent on an individual's abstinence from a target drug or behavior. The reinforcement device—often cash payments, vouchers, or prizes—is contingent on an objective measure of a predetermined therapeutic target. An objective measure often means a biochemical measure, such as urine toxicology testing or the measurement of breath alcohol or carbon monoxide levels, instead of self-reported compliance, which is not verifiable.

The essential principles of CM, as outlined by Petry (2000, 2001a) are to reinforce the treatment goals in three ways:

- Closely monitoring the target behavior
- Providing tangible, positive reinforcement of the target behavior
- Removing the positive reinforcement when the target behavior does not occur.

CM techniques have been developed and tested in the context of clinical trials and settings, and are a clinically accepted tool in fields such as substance abuse, but they have rarely been implemented on a large scale in the manner of CCT programs.

As with CCTs, CM interventions have been tied to participation and the uptake of services in several domains, although risk behaviors are the important determinant for participant selection, rather than income constraints. CM has been shown to improve attendance at HIV drop-in center activities (Petry and others 2001a) and antiviral medication adherence (Rosen and others 2007); drug abuse outcomes (Rawson and others 2002) and uptake rates of counseling sessions (Petry and others 2001b); attendance at weight loss sessions; and attendance in smoking cessation clinics (for example, Emont and Cummings 1992; Higgins and others 1994; Petry 2000). Of particular interest, however, is the use of CM to elicit a complex behavioral change—usually to discourage an unhealthy behavior by positively reinforcing its cessation. Accordingly, the conceptual basis of CM and CCTs is largely similar, although advocates of CM impose no a priori assumptions about the effectiveness of the use of cash as the incentive or reinforcement device, and they have experimented with a variety of reward mechanisms, including vouchers and prizes. In addition, many CM studies are designed to explore effect differences due to variations in the value of the conditionality (known as the "dose-response" curve), the frequency of monitoring and payments, and the length of time that the elicited behavior change is sustained after the program has ended.

Contingency management and substance abuse

The use of CM has been most intensively studied in relation to its efficacy in treating substance abuse. A landmark study by Higgins and others (1994) demonstrated that incentives delivered contingent on submitting cocaine-free urine specimens significantly improved treatment outcomes in ambulatory cocaine-dependent patients. Over 50 percent in the treatment group achieved at least two months of cocaine abstinence versus only 15 percent of the controls. Silverman and others (1996) showed that 47 percent of cocaine-abusing methadone patients assigned to the CM group achieved more than seven weeks of continuous abstinence, compared to only 6 percent of patients in the control group who achieved more than two weeks of abstinence. Similar results have been found for treating opioid dependency (Petry 2000). While CM has also been shown to be efficacious in treating alcohol abuse, the studies are fewer in number due to the difficulties associated with objectively verifying abstinence. Breath, urine, and blood tests can detect alcohol use only up to four to eight hours, which means that effective monitoring would have to take place two or three times a day (Stitzer and Petry 2006).

Contingency management and smoking
Financial incentives to discourage smoking have also been extensively studied. Donatelle and others (2000) used social support and financial incentives to induce high-risk pregnant smokers to quit during their pregnancies. They provided incentives in the amount of US$50 per month for each month of abstinence (up to a maximum of 10 months, which included two months postpartum). Laboratory-verified abstinence was required, and the biochemically confirmed quit rates within the treatment group were higher, both at eight months and two months postpartum. Stitzer and Bigelow (1983) experimented with different levels of cash payment, providing a payment of US$1, $5, or $10 per day for 10 days to the three treatment groups; the control group received no cash. The study found that carbon monoxide levels decreased in an orderly fashion as the payment increased. However, another study by Windsor, Lowe, and Bartlett (1988), which provided cash payments of US$25 at six weeks and six months as a reward for abstinence, found no difference in cessation rates between the control and treatment groups. Other earlier studies experimenting with prizes, vouchers, and in-kind gifts of free nicotine patches showed mixed results, but even positive results disappeared after six months. More recently, Volpp and others (2009) found that while an incentive program's effects on smoking cessation also declined after withdrawal of the incentives, significant effects did still remain three to six months later.

Contingency management and obesity
The use of financial incentives to treat obesity has also gained in popularity, but the evidence regarding efficacy is decidedly more mixed (see Follick, Fowler, and Brown 1984; Jeffery, Thompson, and Wing 1978; and Jeffery

and others 1984). Volpp and others (2008) found significant weight loss from a lottery-based incentive program, but they were not sustained four months after the program's end; similarly, John and others (2011) found matched commitment contracts led to significant weight loss after 36 weeks; again, it was not sustained during a 32-week post-incentive period. A recent systematic review of randomized controlled trials of treatments for obesity (Paul-Ebhohimhen and Avenell 2007) showed no significant effect of the use of financial incentives on weight loss or maintenance at 12 months and 18 months. However, further subanalysis indicated that large transfers (greater than 1.2 percent of personal disposable income) had greater impact, as did rewards for behavioral change rather than weight loss per se and rewards based on group performance rather than individual results. This last point is confirmed by a recent study in the United States that concluded that group-based incentives for weight loss had an impact and that its impact was larger than individual-based incentives (Kullgren and others 2013).

The CM literature, overall, offers useful insights into aspects of the conditionality that appear to elicit the desired behavior change. This is an important area of inquiry that has not been sufficiently explored within CCT programs. However, unlike CCT programs, studies of CM have remained largely experimental and have not been brought to scale (Kane and others 2004; Petry 2000). A recent exception of the financial rewards for weight loss program reported by Cawley and Price (2011, 2013) found high attrition and smaller effects than in the pilot programs. Furthermore, the small sample sizes of study groups—most typically involving groups of 20 to 100, and rarely more than 500—have made it difficult to detect effects that are statistically significant, much less to estimate effect sizes accurately. Also, factorial designs with several treatment arms are common; that—in combination with already small sample sizes—has led to even more constraints on power (Kane and others 2004).

Commitment Devices

If individuals put too much weight on the present when they evaluate the costs and benefits of a decision, they display time-inconsistent preferences. This might be the case when they indulge in instant gratification such as risky sex, overeating, or tobacco, alcohol, or drug consumption. If asked about future choices, they would say, based on their own cost-benefit evaluation, that they would choose the safe behavior. But in the present, they would choose the risky behavior, putting a lot of weight on the instant pleasure and less on the future negative consequences.

Commitment devices are designed to overcome this tendency to be inconsistent over time. Agents enter into these arrangements that restrict their future choice sets by making certain choices more expensive. The arrangements satisfy two conditions: (a) the agents, on the margin, pay something in the present to make those choices more expensive, even if they receive no other benefit for the payment; and (b) the arrangement is individual and does not have a strategic purpose to influence others (Bryan, Karlan, and Nelson 2010). Tirole and Bénabou (2004) develop a theory of internal commitments based on self-reputation over one's willpower, which transforms lapses into precedents that undermine future self-restraint.

Most commitment devices use money to incentivize the behaviors. However, bariatric surgery, which prevents people from eating more in the future or Antabuse or Disulfiram, a drug taken in the morning that makes people sick if they consume alcohol later in the day, are non-monetary examples. The principles behind commitment devices are similar to those at play with CCT and CM; the difference is that individuals pledge their *own* money up front, as a deposit, and only get it back if they satisfy the condition. Commitment devices are a clear acknowledgment of bounded rationality in the behavioral economics framework.

The evidence from commitment devices experiment suggests stronger impacts for smoking cessation than for weight loss. Giné, Karlan, and Zinman (2010) designed and tested a voluntary commitment contract to help smokers in the Philippines to quit smoking. The intervention offered them the opportunity to voluntarily sign a commitment contract to stop smoking. Smokers signing the contract pledged their own money that they would be negative in a urine test detecting nicotine and cotinine six months later. After the commitment period, the participants who passed the urine test got their money back (no interest accrued on the account). If they failed the test, the bank donated the money to charity. The participants who were randomly offered the commitment contract were 3.4 to 5.7 percentage points more likely to pass a urine test for short-term smoking cessation than the control group. This effect persisted in surprise tests at 12 months, indicating that the commitment device produced lasting smoking cessation. These results are consistent with the findings from Gruber and Mullainathan (2005) suggesting that tobacco taxation might make smokers happier, since they value it as an effective commitment device.

Commitment devices have also been tested to encourage weight loss in the United Sates; the evidence is somewhat mixed. Volpp and others (2008) found that a deposit contract incentivized about half of the participants in reaching a target weight loss of 16 pounds, an effect similar to lottery incentives and higher than the 10 percent in the control group. Cawley and Price (2011, 2013) find only modest weight loss from financial incentives for weight loss, but they note that participants in the group who posted forfeitable bonds experienced the largest weight loss. Finally, Burger and Lynham (2010) examine the outcome of weight loss betting markets. This is a type of commitment device whereby individuals bet on their own weight loss. It turns out that most people (80 percent) lost their bet and could not achieve the weight loss they had predicted, despite the money they had gambled on their own performance. Earlier results (Follick, Fowler, and Brown 1984; Jeffery, Thompson, and Wing 1978) also suggest that commitment devices directly linked to weight loss rather than to attendance to weight loss sessions are more effective. Finally it should be noted that there is no evidence on the long-term impacts of such commitment devices.

Subsidies and Loans

Subsidies or subsidized loans are often used to encourage a behavior with positive consequences or externalities. For example, some health insurance companies offer premium reductions for members who engage in activities that can be beneficial for their health, such as membership in a gym. Most risky behaviors have negative consequences or externalities so they are usually taxed rather than subsidized, but prevention methods might be subsidized. The most obvious cases are the free or subsidized distribution of condoms to prevent the spread of HIV/AIDS. Bhatia and others (2005) and Meekers, Agha, and Klein (2005) find increases in condom use in India and Cameroon, respectively, after condom promotion campaigns that included the distribution of free condoms. One limitation of those results, however, is that condom use is self-reported and might be affected by social desirability bias linked to the promotion campaigns. Overall, there is limited evidence about the impact of free condom distribution, whereas the enforcement of the 100 percent condom policy in the sex industry in Thailand seems to have been more successful (Hanenberg and others 1994).

Conclusions and Orientation for Future Research

Tax policies have been shown to be effective as instruments to prevent smoking and alcohol consumption. Most of the evidence comes from developed countries, but an emerging literature from developing countries points in the same direction. As more developing countries adopt and rely more heavily on this policy instrument, additional rigorous evidence should be gathered. The current evidence, however, suggests that substitution effects are usually large. This is well documented for alcohol but is also a factor for tobacco (cigarettes versus other types of tobacco). Potential substitution effects, therefore, need to be taken into account when devising taxation policy.

There is some evidence that the effects of taxation might be different among youth (youth appear to be less responsive to tobacco taxes but more responsive to alcohol taxes). This finding points to the importance of measuring the long-term impacts of the taxation policies. The price elasticity of smoking is generally estimated to be lower in the short run than in the long run, suggesting that it takes time for addicted smokers to adapt to the new price. For alcohol, however, the evidence is more mixed, with diverging results on whether heavy drinkers are more responsive to tax changes.

The evidence is also more mixed for recent experiments in taxing unhealthy food. The very strong substitution effects across food products might be one explanation. Obesity is the result of complex behaviors that are linked not only to food consumption, but also to lack of exercise and a sedentary lifestyle. As such, raising the tax on some unhealthy food might not be sufficient. Finally, the so-called "fat tax" experiences have usually used relatively low tax rates, which might have been insufficient. But the situation is complicated by the fact that—compared to tobacco, alcohol, and drugs—people cannot live without eating and the less healthy food products are often the most affordable for the poor. Nevertheless, as the obesity epidemic is growing and spreading globally, pushes to tax unhealthy food are likely to continue. Those attempts and experiments should be rigorously evaluated to draw lessons about their design and efficacy.

For the other behaviors, such as drug consumption, tax policies are less recommended, either because the behavior is illegal (drugs) or it is difficult to tax (risky sex), or because the limited experiences in taxing it have not been successful so far (unhealthy diet). Approaches relying on information and regulation, covered in the previous chapter, might be the most effective policies to prevent drug use, unhealthy eating, and risky sex, even though experiments with CCTs, CM, and commitment devices should be further encouraged and tested to see if economic incentives could be added to the policy tools for prevention.

In contrast with taxation, developing countries have been leaders in using CCTs and other financial incentives as mechanisms to elicit socially desirable behaviors. They have also experimented with conditional cash transfers to prevent HIV and STIs in Lesotho, Malawi, Mexico, and Tanzania, and with commitment devices to reduce smoking in the Philippines. Those pilot experiments, like many of the contingency management experiments for weight loss and drug use and smoking cessation in richer countries, also integrate recent advances in behavioral economics, using commitment devices that might overcome time inconsistencies or lotteries that might be more appealing to individuals attracted by risk. This line of research should be encouraged, since it would help to assess the contribution of nudge and choice architecture interventions to the improvement of health outcomes.

As those prevention designs that rely on financial incentives are further evaluated and potentially scaled up, they might usefully be integrated with more traditional CCTs aimed at providing a consumption floor for poor households and at increasing school participation and health care visits. From an operational point of view, this integration would allow those incentive mechanisms to reach a large segment of the population.

Experiments testing financial incentive mechanisms should try to systematically test the existence of long-term or sustained impacts, since those are the most relevant for public health. In any case, for all the behaviors covered in this volume, economic mechanisms, in the form of taxes or other types of financial incentives, should go hand in hand with continued information campaigns and government regulation.

Notes

1. In the United States, the evidence is more mixed on the impact of price and taxes on smoking among youth (DeCicca, Kenkel, and Mathios 2002, 2008; Ross and Chaloupka 2003). Generally, the effect of tax increases is larger on smoking cessation than on smoking initiation.
2. See Cawley (2012) for a review; also see Chouinard and others (2007); Fletcher and others (2010a, 2010b); Gelbach, Klick, and Stratmann (2009); and Schroeter, Lusk, and Tyner (2008) for specific studies.

References

Baird, Sarah, Ephraim Chirwa, Craig McIntosh, and Berk Özler. 2010. "The Short-Term Impacts of a Schooling Conditional Cash Transfer Program on the Sexual Behavior of Young Women." *Health Economics* 19 (S1): 55–68. doi:10.1002/hec.1569.

Baird, Sarah, Richard Garfein, Craig McIntosh, and Berk Özler. 2012. "Impact of a Cash Transfer Program for Schooling on Prevalence of HIV and HSV-2 in Malawi: A Cluster Randomized Trial." *Lancet* 379 (9823): 1320–29. doi:10.1016/S0140-6736(11)61709-1.

Bellis, Mark A., Karen Hughes, Michela Morleo, Karen Tocque, Sara Hughes, Tony Allen, Dominic Harrison, and Eduardo Fe-Rodriguez. 2007. "Predictors of Risky Alcohol Consumption in Schoolchildren and Their Implications for Preventing Alcohol-Related Harm." *Substance Abuse Treatment, Prevention, and Policy* 2: 15.

Bhatia, V., H. M. Swami, A. Parashar, and T. R. Justin. 2005. "Condom-Promotion Programme among Slum-Dwellers in Chandigarh, India." *Public Health* 119 (5): 382–84.

Bird, Richard M., and Sally Wallace. 2010. "Taxing Alcohol in Africa: Reflections and Updates." Working Paper 1031, International Center for Public Policy, Andrew Young School of Policy Studies, Georgia State University, Atlanta.

Björkman-Nyqvist, Martina, Lucia Corno, Damien de Walque, and Jakob Svensson. 2013. "HIV Prevention: Evidence from a Randomized Field Experiment on Lottery Incentives." Unpublished manuscript.

Booth, Andrew, Petra Meier, Tim Stockwell, Anthea Sutton, Anna Wilkinson, Ruth Wong, Alan Brennan, Daragh O'Reilly, Robin Purshouse, and Karl Taylor. 2008. "Independent Review of the Effects of Alcohol Pricing and Promotion." Project Report for the Department of Health, University of Sheffield, South Yorkshire, U.K. http://www.sheffield.ac.uk/scharr/sections/ph/research/alpol/publications.

Bryan, Gharad, Dean Karlan, and Scott Nelson. 2010. "Commitment Devices." *Annual Review of Economics* 2: 671–98.

Burger, Nicholas, and John Lynham. 2010. "Betting on Weight Loss … and Losing: Personal Gambles as Commitment Mechanisms." *Applied Economics Letters* 17 (12): 1161–66.

Cawley, John. 2012. "Taxes on Energy Dense Foods to Improve Nutrition and Prevent Obesity." In *Food and Addiction: A Comprehensive Handbook*, edited by Kelly D. Brownell and Mark S. Gold, 439–49. New York: Oxford University Press.

Cawley, John, and Joshua A. Price. 2011. "Outcomes in a Program That Offers Financial Rewards for Weight Loss." In *Economic Aspects of Obesity*, edited by Michael Grossman and Naci Mocan, 91–126. Chicago: National Bureau of Economic Research and University of Chicago Press.

———. 2013. "A Case Study of a Workplace Wellness Program That Offers Financial Incentives for Weight Loss." *Journal of Health Economics* 32 (5): 794–805.

Chaloupka, Frank J., Michael Grossman, and Henry Saffer. 2002. "The Effects of Price on Alcohol Consumption and Alcohol-Related Problems." *Alcohol Research and Health* 26 (1): 22–34.

Chaloupka, Frank J., Teh-wei Hu, Kenneth E. Warner, Rowena Jacobs, and Ayda Yurekli. 2000. "The Taxation of Tobacco Products." In *Economics of Tobacco Control: Tobacco Control in Developing Countries*, edited by Prabhat Jha and Frank J. Chaloupka, 237–72. Oxford, U.K.: Oxford University Press.

Chaloupka, Frank J., and Adit Laixuthai. 1997. "Do Youths Substitute Alcohol and Marijuana? Some Econometric Evidence." *Eastern Economic Journal* 23 (3): 253–76.

Chaloupka, Frank J., Henry Saffer, and Michael Grossman. 1993. "Alcohol-Control Policies and Motor-Vehicle Fatalities." *Journal of Legal Studies* 22 (1): 161–86.

Chouinard, Hayley H., David E. Davis, Jeffrey T. LaFrance, and Jeffrey M. Perloff. 2007. "Fat Taxes: Big Money for Small Change." *Forum for Health Economics & Policy* 10 (2): 1–30.

Claro, Rafael M., Renata B. Levy, Barry M. Popkin, and Carlos A. Monteiro. 2012. "Sugar-Sweetened Beverage Taxes in Brazil." *American Journal of Public Health* 102 (1): 178–83.

Cook, Philip J., and George Tauchen. 1982. "The Effect of Liquor Taxes on Heavy Drinking." *Bell Journal of Economics* 13 (2): 379–90.

DeCicca, Philip, Donald Kenkel, and Alan D. Mathios. 2002. "Putting Out the Fires: Will Higher Taxes Reduce the Onset of Youth Smoking?" *Journal of Political Economy* 110 (1): 144–69.

———. 2008. "Cigarette Taxes and the Transition from Youth to Adult Smoking: Smoking Initiation, Cessation, and Participation." *Journal of Health Economics* 27 (4): 904–17.

DeSimone, Jeff, and Matthew C. Farrelly. 2003. "Price and Enforcement Effects on Cocaine and Marijuana Demand." *Economic Inquiry* 41 (1): 98–115.

de Walque, Damien, William H. Dow, Rose Nathan, Ramadhani Abdul, Faraji Abilahi, Erick Gong, Zachary Isdahl, Julian Jamison, Boniphace Jullu, Suneeta Krishnan, Albert Majura, Edward Miguel, Jeanne Moncada, Sally Mtenga, Mathew Alexander Mwanyangala, Laura Packel, Julius Schachter, Kizito Shirima, and Carol A. Medlin. 2012. "Incentivizing Safe Sex: A Randomized Trial of Conditional Cash Transfers for HIV and Sexually Transmitted Infection Prevention in Rural Tanzania." *British Medical Journal Open* 2:e000747. doi:10.1136/bmjopen-2011-000747.

de Walque, Damien, William H. Dow, Carol Medlin, and Rose Nathan. 2012. "Stimulating Demand for AIDS Prevention: Lessons from the RESPECT Trial." Policy Research Working Paper 5973, World Bank, Washington, DC.

Donatelle, Rebecca J., Susan L. Prows, Donna Champeau, and Deanne Hudson. 2000. "Randomised Controlled Trial Using Social Support and Financial Incentives for High Risk Pregnant Smokers: Significant Other Supporter (SOS) Program." *Tobacco Control* 9 (S3): 11167–69.

Emont, Seth L., and K. Michael Cummings. 1992. "Using a Low-Cost, Prize-Drawing Incentive to Improve Recruitment Rate at a Work-Site Smoking Cessation Clinic." *Journal of Occupational Medicine* 34 (8): 771–74.

Evans, William N., and Jeanne S. Ringel. 1999. "Can Higher Cigarette Taxes Improve Birth Outcomes?" *Journal of Public Economics* 72 (1): 135–54.

Faulkner, Guy E. J., Paul Grootendorst, Van Hai Nguyen, Tatiana Andreyeva, Kelly Arbour-Nicitopoulos, M. Christopher Auld, Sean B. Cash, John Cawley, Peter Donnelly, Adam Drewnowski, Laurette Dubé, Roberta Ferrence, Ian Janssen, Jeffrey LaFrance, Darius Lakdawalla, Rena Mendelsen, Lisa M. Powell, W. Bruce Traill, and Frank Windmeijer. 2011. "Economic Instruments for Obesity Prevention: Results of a Scoping Review and Modified Delphi Survey." *International Journal of Behavioral Nutrition and Physical Activity* 8: 109.

Fernald, Lisa C. H., Paul J. Gertler, and Xiaohui Hou. 2008. "Cash Component of Conditional Cash Transfer Program Is Associated with Higher Body Mass Index and Blood Pressure in Adults." *Journal of Nutrition* 138 (11): 2250–57.

Fernald, Lisa C. H., Paul H. Gertler, and Lynnette M. Neufeld. 2008. "Role of Cash in Conditional Cash Transfer Programmes for Child Health, Growth, and Development: An Analysis of Mexico's Oportunidades." *Lancet* 371 (9615): 827–37.

Finkelstein, Eric A., Laura A. Linnan, Deborah F. Tate, and Ben E. Birken. 2007. "A Pilot Study Testing the Effect of Different Levels of Financial Incentives on Weight Loss among Overweight Employees." *Journal of Occupational and Environmental Medicine* 49 (9): 981–89.

Fletcher, Jason M., David E. Frisvold, and Nathan Tefft. 2010a. "Can Soft Drink Taxes Reduce Population Weight?" *Contemporary Economic Policy* 28 (1): 23–35.

———. 2010b. "The Effects of Soft Drink Taxes on Child and Adolescent Consumption and Weight Outcomes." *Journal of Public Economics* 94 (11–12): 967–74.

Follick, Michael J., Joanne L. Fowler, and Richard A. Brown. 1984. "Attrition in Worksite Weight-Loss Interventions: The Effects of an Incentive Procedure." *Journal of Consultative Clinical Psychology* 52 (1): 139–40.

Galárraga, Omar, Sandra G. Sosa-Rubi, César Infante, Paul J. Gertler, and Stefano M. Bertozzi. 2013. "Willingness-to-Accept Reduction in HIV Risks: Conditional Economic Incentives in Mexico." *European Journal of Health Economics* 2 (2): 1–15.

Gallet, Craig A. 2007. "The Demand for Alcohol: A Meta-analysis of Elasticities." *Australian Journal of Agricultural and Resource Economics* 51 (2): 121–35.

Gallet, Craig A., and John A. List. 2003. "Cigarette Demand: A Meta-analysis of Elasticities." *Health Economics* 12 (10): 821–35.

Gelbach, Jonah B., Jonathan Klick, and Thomas Stratmann. 2009. "Cheap Donuts and Expensive Broccoli: The Effect of Relative Prices on Obesity." *Contemporary Economic Policy* 28 (1): 23–35.

Gertler, Paul. 2004. "Do Conditional Cash Transfers Improve Child Health? Evidence from PROGRESA's Control Randomized Experiment." *American Economic Review* 94 (2): 332–41.

Gertler, Paul, Manisha Shah, and Stefano M. Bertozzi. 2005. "Risky Business: The Market for Unprotected Sex." *Journal of Political Economy* 113 (3): 518–50.

Giné, Xavier, Dean Karlan, and Jonathan Zinman. 2010. "Put Your Money Where Your Butt Is: A Commitment Contract for Smoking Cessation." *American Economic Journal: Applied Economics* 2 (4): 213–35.

Grossman, Michael. 1993. "The Economic Analysis of Addictive Behavior." In *Economics and the Prevention of Alcohol-Related Problems*, edited by Michael E. Hilton and Gregory Bloss, 91–123. Research Monograph 25, Pub. No. 93–3513. Bethesda, MD: National Institute on Alcohol Abuse and Alcoholism.

Gruber, Jonathan H., and Sendhil Mullainathan. 2005. "Do Cigarette Taxes Make Smokers Happier?" *Advances in Economic Analysis & Policy* 5 (1): 1–43.

Gruenewald, Paul J., William R. Ponicki, Harold D. Holder, and Anders Romelsjö. 2006. "Alcohol Prices, Beverage Quality, and the Demand for Alcohol: Quality Substitutions and Price Elasticities." *Alcoholism: Clinical and Experimental Research* 30 (1): 96–105.

Guindon, G. Emmanuel, Anne-Marie Perucic, and David Boisclair. 2003. "Higher Tobacco Prices and Taxes in South-East Asia." Health, Nutrition, and Population Discussion Paper 11, World Bank, Washington, DC.

Hanenberg, Robert S., Wiwat Rojanapithayakorn, Prayura Kunasol, and David C. Sokal. 1994. "Impact of Thailand's HIV-Control Programme as Indicated by the Decline of Sexually Transmitted Diseases." *Lancet* 344 (8917): 243–45.

Hidayat, Budi, and Hasbullah Thabrany. 2010. "Cigarette Smoking in Indonesia: Examination of a Myopic Model of Addictive Behaviour." *International Journal of Environmental Research in Public Health* 7 (6): 2473–85.

Higgins, Stephen T., Alan J. Budney, Warren K. Bickel, Florian E. Foerg, Robert Donham, and Gary J. Badger. 1994. "Incentives Improve Outcome in Outpatient Behavioral Treatment of Cocaine Dependence." *Archives of General Psychiatry* 51 (7): 568–76.

Hu, Teh-wei, Zhengzhong Mao, Jian Shi, and Wendong Chen. 2010. "The Role of Taxation in Tobacco Control and Its Potential Economic Impact in China." *Tobacco Control* 19 (1): 58–64.

Jeffery, Robert W., Wendy M. Bjornson-Benson, Barbara S. Rosenthal, Candace L. Kurth, and Mary M. Dunn. 1984. "Effectiveness of Monetary Contracts with

Two Repayment Schedules of Weight Reduction in Men and Women from Self-Referred and Population Samples." *Behavioral Therapy* 15 (3): 273–79.

Jeffery, Robert W., Paul D. Thompson, and Rena R. Wing. 1978. "Effects on Weight Reduction of Strong Monetary Contracts for Calorie Restriction or Weight Loss." *Behaviour Research and Therapy* 16 (5): 363–69.

John, Leslie K., George Loewenstein, Andrea B. Troxel, Laurie Norton, Jennifer E. Fassbender, and Kevin G. Volpp. 2011. "Financial Incentives for Extended Weight Loss: A Randomized, Controlled Trial." *Journal of General Internal Medicine* 26 (6): 621–26.

Kane, Robert L., Paul E. Johnson, Robert J. Town, and Mary Butler. 2004. "A Structured Review of the Effect of Economic Incentives on Consumers' Preventive Behavior." *American Journal of Preventive Medicine* 27 (4): 327–52.

Kenkel, Donald S. 2005. "Are Alcohol Tax Hikes Fully Passed through to Prices? Evidence from Alaska." *American Economic Review* 95 (2): 273–77.

Kohler, Hans-Peter, and Rebecca L. Thornton. 2011. "Conditional Cash Transfers and HIV/AIDS Prevention: Unconditionally Promising?" *World Bank Economic Review* 26 (2): 165–90. doi: 10.1093/wber/lhr041.

Kullgren, Jeffrey T., Andrea B. Toxel, George Loewenstein, David A. Asch, Lisa Wesby, Tao Yuanyun, Zhu Jingsan, and Kevin G. Volpp. 2013. "Individual-Versus Group-Based Financial Incentives for Weight Loss: A Randomized, Controlled Trial." *Annals of Internal Medicine* 158 (7): 505–14.

Kuo, Meichun, Jean-Luc Heeb, Gerhard Gmel, and Jürgen Rehm. 2003. "Does Price Matter? The Effect of Decreased Price on Spirits Consumption in Switzerland." *Alcoholism: Clinical and Experimental Research* 27 (4): 720–25.

Lagarde, Mylene, Andy Haines, and Natasha Palmer. 2007. "Conditional Cash Transfers for Improving Uptake of Health Interventions in Low- and Middle-Income Countries: A Systematic Review." *Journal of the American Medical Society* 298 (16): 1900–10.

Lance, Peter M., John S. Akin, William H. Dow, and Chung-Ping Loh. 2004. "Is Cigarette Smoking in Poorer Nations Highly Sensitive to Price? Evidence from Russia and China." *Journal of Health Economics* 23 (1): 173–89.

Levy, Douglas E., and Ellen Meara. 2006. "The Effect of the 1998 Master Settlement Agreement on Prenatal Smoking." *Journal of Health Economics* 25 (2): 276–94.

Manning, Willard G., Linda Blumberg, and Lawrence H. Moulton. 1995. "The Demand for Alcohol: The Differential Response to Price. *Journal of Health Economics* 14 (2): 123–48.

Medlin, Carol, and Damien de Walque. 2008. "Potential Applications of Conditional Cash Transfers for Prevention of Sexually Transmitted Infections and HIV in Sub-Saharan Africa." Policy Research Working Paper 4673, World Bank, Washington, DC.

Meekers, Dominique, Sohail Agha, and Megan Klein. 2005. "The Impact on Condom Use of the '100% Jeune' Social Marketing Program in Cameroon." *Journal of Adolescent Health* 36 (6): 530.

Moore, Michael J. 1996. "Death and Tobacco Taxes." *RAND Journal of Economics* 27 (2): 415–28.

Müller, Stefanie, Daniela Piontek, Alexander Pabst, Sebastian E. Baumeister, and Ludwig Kraus. 2010. "Changes in Alcohol Consumption and Beverage

Preference among Adolescents after the Introduction of the Alcopops Tax in Germany." *Addiction* 105 (7): 1205–13.

Mytton, Oliver T., Dushy Clarke, and Mike Rayner. 2012. "Taxing Unhealthy Food and Drinks to Improve Health." *British Medical Journal* 344: e2931–e2931.

Nelson, Jon P. 2008. "How Similar Are Youth and Adult Alcohol Behaviors? Panel Results for Excise Taxes and Outlet Density." *Atlantic Economic Journal* 36 (1): 89–104.

Ng, Shu W., Fengying Zhai, and Barry M. Popkin. 2008. "Impacts of China's Edible Oil Pricing Policy on Nutrition. *Social Science & Medicine* 66 (2): 414–26.

Ohsfeldt, Robert L., and Michael A. Morrisey. 1997. "Beer Taxes, Workers' Compensation, and Industrial Injury." *Review of Economics and Statistics* 79 (1): 155–60.

Okello, Andrew K. 2001. "An Analysis of Excise Taxation in Kenya." African Economic Policy Discussion Paper 73, Belfer Center for Science and International Affairs, Harvard University, Cambridge, MA.

Paul-Ebhohimhen, Virginia, and Alison Avenell. 2007. "Systematic Review of the Use of Financial Incentive in Treatments for Obesity and Overweight." *Obesity Reviews* 9 (4): 355–67.

Petry, Nancy M. 2000. "A Comprehensive Guide to the Application of Contingency Management Procedures in Clinical Settings." *Drug and Alcohol Dependence* 58 (1–2): 9–25.

Petry, Nancy M., Bonnie Martin, and Charles Finocche. 2001a. "Contingency Management in Group Treatment: A Demonstration Project in an HIV Drop-In Center." *Journal of Substance Abuse Treatment* 21 (2): 89–96.

Petry, Nancy M., Ismene Petrakis, Louis Trevisan, George Wiredu, Nashaat N. Boutros, Bonnie Martin, and Thomas R. Kosten. 2001b. "Contingency Management Interventions: From Research to Practice." *American Journal of Psychiatry* 158 (5): 694–702.

Powell, Lisa M., and Frank J. Chaloupka. 2009. "Food Prices and Obesity: Evidence and Policy Implications for Taxes and Subsidies." *Milbank Quarterly* 87 (1): 229–57.

Ramful, Preety, and Xuey Zhao. 2008. "Individual Heterogeneity in Alcohol Consumption: The Case of Beer, Wine and Spirits in Australia." *Economic Record* 84 (265): 207–22.

Rao, Vijayendra, Indrani Gupta, Michael Lokshin, and Smarajit Jana. 2003. "Sex Workers and the Cost of Safe Sex: The Compensating Differential for Condom Use among Calcutta Prostitutes." *Journal of Development Economics* 71 (2): 585–603.

Rawson, Richard A., Alice Huber, Michael McCann, Steven Shoptaw, David Farabee, Chris Reiber, and Walter Ling. 2002. "A Comparison of Contingency Management and Cognitive-Behavioral Approaches during Methadone Maintenance Treatment for Cocaine Dependence." *Archives of General Psychiatry* 59 (9): 817–24.

Rosen, Marc I., Kevin Dieckhaus, Thomas J. McMahon, Barbara Valdes, Nancy M. Petry, Joyce Cramer, and Bruce Rounsaville. 2007. "Improved Adherence with Contingency Management." *AIDS Patient Care STDS* 21 (1): 30–40.

Ross, Hana, and Frank J. Chaloupka. 2003. "The Effect of Cigarette Prices on Youth Smoking." *Health Economics* 12 (3): 217–30.

Ruhm, Christopher J. 1996. "Alcohol Policies and Highway Vehicle Fatalities." *Journal of Health Economics* 15 (4): 435–54.

Saffer, Henry, and Michael Grossman. 1987. "Beer Taxes, the Legal Drinking Age, and Youth Motor Vehicle Fatalities." *Journal of Legal Studies* 16 (2): 351–74.

Schroeter, Christiane, Jayson Lusk, and Wallace Tyner. 2008. "Determining the Impact of Food Price and Income Changes on Body Weight." *Journal of Health Economics* 27 (1): 45–68.

Silverman, Kenneth, Stephen T. Higgins, Robert K. Brooner, Ivan D. Montoya, Edward J. Cone, Charles R. Schuster, and Kenzie L. Preston. 1996. "Sustained Cocaine Abstinence in Methodone-Maintenance Patients through Voucher-Based Reinforcement Therapy." *Archives of General Psychiatry* 53 (5): 409–15.

Sloan, Frank A., Bridget A. Reilly, and Christoph Schenzler. 1994. "Effects of Prices, Civil and Criminal Sanctions, and Law Enforcement on Alcohol-Related Mortality." *Journal of Studies on Alcohol* 55 (4): 454–65.

Stitzer, Maxine L., and George E. Bigelow. 1983. "Contingent Payment for Carbon Monoxide Reduction: Effects of Pay Amount." *Behavioral Therapy* 14 (2): 647–56.

Stitzer, Maxine L., and Nancy Petry. 2006. "Contingency Management for Treatment of Substance Abuse." *Annual Review of Clinical Psychology* 2: 411–34.

Thornton, Rebecca L. 2008. "The Demand for and Impact of Learning HIV Status." *American Economic Review* 98 (5): 1829–63.

Tirole, Jean, and Roland Bénabou. 2004. "Willpower and Personal Rules." *Journal of Political Economy* 112 (4): 848–86.

Treisman, Daniel. 2010. "Death and Prices: The Political Economy of Russia's Alcohol Crisis." *Economics of Transition* 18 (2): 281–331.

Volpp, Kevin G., Leslie K. John, Andrea B. Troxel, Laurie Norton, Jennifer Fassbender, and George Lowenstein. 2008. "Financial Incentive-Based Approaches for Weight Loss: A Randomized Trial." *Journal of the American Medical Association* 300 (22): 2631–37.

Volpp, Kevin G., Andrea B. Troxel, Mark V. Pauly, Henry A. Glick, Andrea Puig, David A. Asch, Robert Galvin, Jingsan Zhu, Fei Wan, Jill DeGuzman, Elizabeth Corbett, Janet Weiner, and Janet Audrain-McGovern. 2009. "A Randomized Controlled Trial of Financial Incentives for Smoking Cessation." *New England Journal of Medicine* 360: 699–709.

Wagenaar, Alexander C., Matthew J. Salois, and Kelli A. Komro. 2009. "Effects of Beverage Alcohol Price and Tax Levels on Drinking: A Meta-Analysis of 1,003 Estimates from 112 Studies." *Addiction* 104 (2): 179–90.

Williams, Jenny, Frank J. Chaloupka, and Henry Wechsler. 2005. "Are There Differential Effects of Price and Policy on College Students' Drinking Intensity?" *Contemporary Economic Policy* 23 (1): 78–90.

Windsor, Richard A., John B. Lowe, and Edward E. Bartlett. 1988. "The Effectiveness of a Worksite Self-Help Smoking Cessation Program: A Randomized Trial." *Journal of Behavioral Medicine* 11 (4): 407–21.

Young, Douglas J., and Agnieszka Bielinska-Kwapisz. 2006. "Alcohol Prices, Consumption, and Traffic Fatalities." *Southern Economic Journal* 72 (3): 690–703.

Zulfiqar, Ali, Atiur Rahman, and Taifur Rahman. 2003. "Appetite for Nicotine: An Economic Analysis of Tobacco Control in Bangladesh." Health, Nutrition, and Policy Discussion Paper 16, World Bank, Washington, DC.

6

Conclusions

Damien de Walque

All over the world, individuals engage in behaviors that are risky for their health. They smoke, use illicit drugs, drink too much alcohol, eat unhealthy food or adopt sedentary lifestyles, and have risky sexual encounters. As a consequence, they endanger their health, reduce their own life expectancy, and often impose consequences on others. All of these risky behaviors are prevalent in developing countries, and some constitute growing threats for the health of their populations.

Despite recent progress in prevention and treatment, the HIV/AIDS epidemic—one of the most devastating consequences of risky sex—remains a heavy burden in Sub-Saharan Africa, especially in its southern cone; teenage pregnancies continue to jeopardize the health of mothers and children in many countries. Drug and alcohol abuse have been relatively stable over the past decade, but smoking and obesity linked to unhealthy diets are on the rise in many developing countries and have the potential to substantially increase mortality and morbidity.

In contrast with other ailments, all of these risky behaviors are, ultimately, the result of decisions made by individuals. Individuals decide to light a cigarette, consume drugs, order alcoholic drinks, eat junk food, or have unprotected sex. Those decisions, however, are more complex than they may appear. Individuals might be trading their long-term well-being for immediate pleasure. Such trade-offs will depend on prices, information about the health consequences, and their own subjective beliefs. The choice to engage in risky behaviors is affected by how people value their well-being in the future, which in turn is a function of their education, wealth, and competing health risks, that is, other health risks that could affect their well-being or life expectancy. Social norms and the composition of social networks also play roles: by defining how certain behaviors are perceived in a certain network, they might alter the present benefit derived from these behaviors.

Individuals, moreover, differ not only in the costs and benefits they face but also in the way in which they make their decisions. For example, characteristics such as impatience and lack of self-control can make individuals more present-biased and increase their propensity to take risks. There are important differences in the way people respond to external stimuli: addicts react differently than non-addicts, and risk-taking increases in adolescence as a result of changes to the brain around puberty. Understanding the heterogeneity in decision making is crucial to the development of effective prevention programs, but the research on these topics is only emerging and mainly comes from developed countries. This important research gap in developing countries needs to be filled.

Engaging in a risky behavior carries considerable risk of both dying early and living many years with compromised health. The consequent diseases include cancer, AIDS, liver cirrhosis, and diabetes and are expensive to treat, even in low-income, resource-poor settings. They exert a significant toll on individuals' productivity. In most low-income countries, it is difficult to formally insure against these costly consequences, given the rarity of both health insurance and public or private disability benefits. According to the World Bank's World Development Indicators, 75 percent of private expenditure on health was financed through out-of-pocket payments in low-income countries in 2011.

Each of these risky behaviors can also directly influence the health of family members, coworkers, and others in the immediate environments. The immediate peers of those who engage in risky behaviors also experience declines in their productivity. Children might suffer a reduction in the amount invested in their human capital, either because they must forgo schooling due to a sick parent or because exposure in utero has put them on a lower trajectory in terms of cognitive abilities.

Society also loses when individuals engage in behaviors that put their health at risk. While substantial, the opportunity costs of the medical spending required to deal with the resulting diseases are far outweighed by their productivity losses in low-income countries. Moreover, existing studies do not even take into account the future productivity losses associated with the adverse effects that children face when the adults in their lives engage in risky behaviors.

The costly impacts that accrue to individuals in developing countries, in addition to the presence of large spillovers to peers and society, suggest that public intervention to prevent or reduce engagement in these behaviors can improve overall welfare.

Different types of public health interventions are used to prevent risky behaviors: on the one hand are legislation and information, education, and communication (IEC) programs; on the other hand are interventions using price mechanisms, taxes, or financial incentives.

The evidence suggests that legislation tends to be effective, especially when enforcement mechanisms are strong. For example, comprehensive advertising bans on cigarettes were found to be more effective than partial advertising bans (Blecher 2008). Similarly, when the prohibition of alcohol in America in the 1920s and poppy cultivation in Afghanistan in 2001 were both stringently enforced, the uses of both substances decreased sharply. However, in those two cases, the unintended consequences of these policies—namely, the crime surge in the Prohibition era and the brutality of the enforcement under the Taliban in Afghanistan—were especially severe.

In general, IEC programs have been less effective in changing behavior. Calorie labeling laws and school-based sex education programs inform consumers about the risks associated with certain behaviors, but translating that knowledge into concrete behavioral changes seems harder to achieve.

This is not meant to discredit all IEC efforts as ineffective—far from it. As the graphic warnings on cigarettes have shown, IEC messages that are targeted and reinforced at regular intervals can be very effective in changing behavior. It can also be the case that IEC works to influence general societal attitudes toward risk, which are harder to measure and hence harder to demonstrate as effective. IEC is certain to play an important role in changing attitudes and must go hand in hand with any risk behavior change programs.

Tax policies have been shown to be efficient as instruments to prevent smoking and alcohol consumption. Most of the evidence comes from developed countries, but an emerging literature from developing countries points in the same direction. As more developing countries adopt and rely more heavily on this policy instrument, additional rigorous evidence should be collected.

Substitution effects are important to consider when implementing public interventions. Drug legislation provides a good example: opium bans resulted in an increase in the use of heroin. Substitution effects can also be beneficial, as in the legalization of marijuana. In the United States, this legalization resulted in a decrease in the rate of overdose of heroin and opium due to people switching to marijuana (Model 1993); moreover, in a study in the United Kingdom (Adda, McConnel, and Rasul 2011), legalization is linked to a decrease in violent crime, partially due to the freeing up of local police forces from marijuana-related crackdowns.

With taxation, substitution effects are usually substantial. This is well documented for alcohol but is also a factor for different tobacco products. Accordingly, potential substitution effects need to be taken into account when devising taxation policies. The very strong substitution effects across food products might be one explanation for the mixed evidence from recent experiments in taxing unhealthy food.

In contrast to taxation, developing countries have been leaders in using conditional cash transfers and other financial incentives as mechanisms to elicit socially desirable behaviors. They have also experimented with conditional cash transfers to prevent HIV and STIs, or commitment devices to reduce smoking, such as an incentive mechanism whereby individuals commit their own funds up front and forfeit them if they engage in the risky behavior. Those pilot experiments, like many of the contingency management experiments for weight loss and drug use and smoking cessation in richer countries, are integrating recent advances in behavioral economics, using commitment devices that might overcome time inconsistency or lotteries that might be more appealing to individuals attracted by risk. This line of research should be encouraged, since it would help assess the contribution of nudge and choice architecture interventions to improve health outcomes.

In addition to the efficacy and effectiveness of public interventions, the length of their effect is an important question to study. The review of the evidence suggests that even if an intervention is effective, the duration of its effect varies and is a function of the length and intensity with which the intervention was delivered. When the intervention is removed, there is likely to be a "bounce back" effect to levels similar to those before its introduction. This was seen in the United States with the repeal of the prohibition of alcohol, and in Afghanistan with the fall of the Taliban, who had eradicated poppy cultivation.

Even if an intervention is maintained for a long time, its effect can be attenuated. For example, Thailand's 100 percent condom policy in the prostitution sector has been found to be less effective now than it was immediately after enactment. To prevent a similar desensitization, the Framework Convention on Tobacco Control requires that graphic warnings on cigarette boxes be "rotating" so that smokers are continually exposed to new images that will reinforce the message.

It is also important to measure the long-term effects of taxation policies. Some evidence suggests that the effects might be different among youth, who appear to be less responsive to tobacco taxes but more responsive to alcohol taxes. The price elasticity of smoking is generally estimated to be lower in the short term than in the long term, suggesting that it takes time for addicted smokers to adapt to the new price. But for alcohol, the evidence is more mixed, with diverging results on whether heavy drinkers are more responsive to tax changes.

Across risky behaviors, certain enabling conditions emerge that make it more likely for an intervention to be effective: design, targeting, and enforcement. In terms of design, more successful interventions take into account the local culture. Targeting interventions to subpopulations is also important—just because an intervention is not effective in a general population does not necessarily imply that it will not work for specific sub-groups that might be especially vulnerable. Finally, interventions that are supported by a strong enforcement mechanism tend to be more effective.

In terms of research gaps, there is an urgent need to undertake more rigorous experimental and quasi-experimental evaluations of health interventions. Most evaluations consist of post-only designs, or at best, a pre-post design without a control group. This limitation compromises the internal validity of the study and makes it hard to determine causal effects. Including a suitable control group would greatly strengthen the level of evidence and can often be done readily if considered in the design stage.

In terms of geographic spread of evidence, a gap exists in the evidence emerging from low- and middle-income countries. This is often because interventions are being introduced in these countries, which limits the availability of evaluation results. However, prioritizing evaluations from the start would allow the collection of baseline data and selection of controls, which would enable rigorous evaluations to be conducted at later stages. With low- and middle-income countries confronting emerging threats linked to risky behaviors for health, it is even more imperative to generate robust evidence on interventions that work.

References

Adda, Jérôme, Brendon McConnel, and Imran Rasul. 2011. "Crime and the Depenalization of Cannabis Possession: Evidence from a Policing Experiment." Unpublished manuscript, University College London, U.K.

Blecher, E. 2008. "The Impact of Tobacco Advertising Bans on Consumption in Developing Countries." *Journal of Health Economics* 27 (4): 930–42.

Model, Katryn E. 1993. "The Effect of Marijuana Decriminalization on Hospital Emergency Room Drug Episodes: 1975–1978." *Journal of the American Statistical Association* 88 (423): 737–47.

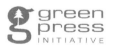